DISCLAIMER: This book is a guide to the practice of Abdominal Acupuncture and all prescriptions and acupuncture point depths are suggestions only and should only be used by qualified acupuncturists. The author and publishers cannot accept any responsibility for any harm or injury that may arise as a result of misuse of the information contained in this book.

Contents

Table of Figures content;

Dedication

I wish to dedicate this book to my mother Maeve, to my beautiful partner Anna Goodere, to my son Conor and daughters Aisling and Keela Shipsey - you all make my life complete.

Preface

I had been in the company of Dr. Han Yan for less than 20 minutes when I realised she was about to change my life. I had been studying at the University of Traditional Chinese Medicine (TCM) Nanjing in China for only a few months when I got the opportunity to do an internship with Dr. Han. I was very excited because I now had the chance to study with a doctor renowned in abdominal acupuncture (AA).

Though a relatively new practice AA was becoming more popular in China back in 2000. In Ireland, however, it was practically unknown. Still, as a student myself I had, during my continued learning, come across reports and revelations about the effectiveness of this system and I was keen to learn more. Now I was here in the bustling clinic in Jiangzu Province Hospital, standing behind the respected doctor as she spoke in rapid Mandarin to a woman crumpled up in pain from a frozen shoulder.

I watched as Dr. Han assessed the patient in the usual way, asking questions, observing the body and taking the distressed woman's pulse. As Dr. Han palpated the patient's abdomen, then measured and marked out the area of attention using her forefinger and thumb as guide and iodine as a visual indicator, she explained to me each step she was taking and why. Needles were inserted at a superficial level. I looked to the woman lying now on the hospital bed but she showed no signs of even noticing that the needles had been introduced.

Dr. Han, her voice instructive but soft so as not to unsettle the patient, listed the points of insertion for my benefit, adjusting them with a swift, elegant sliding motion to reach the correct depths and allow her to disseminate the secrets that lay beneath. In this way, she told me, the needle at the shoulder point and the Ahshi (painful point) were fine tuned.

Dr. Han instructed the patient to move her shoulder, which the woman duly did, a smile of surprise lighting her face as she realised the intense pain had eased somewhat and mobility had increased. Nodding knowingly, Dr. Han adjusted two of the needles, reducing the pain even more.

Inserting a further Ahshi point into the area, the good doctor asked the patient once again to move her shoulder. This time the woman's broad smile was accompanied by a laugh of glee. The pain had completely disappeared and full movement had been restored to the area of her body that minutes before had been aching in agony.

I watched in amazement Dr. Han chuckled both at my bemused face and her patient's excitement. "I knew the last needle would clear the pain," she told me confidently.

I nodded back at her, unable to say anything that could fully encompass what I was feeling at that stage. I had watched acupuncture performed with the delicacy and accuracy of a master calligrapher's brushstroke and I was captivated. The result was as beautiful as a finished ancient artwork and the woman's smile more memorable to me than the *Mona Lisa*. I knew there and then that this was the path my practice would take and that my time with Dr. Han was only the start of a long journey to develop my skills as a specialist in AA.

Ever since that first experience of abdominal acupuncture in September 2000 I have been fascinated and mesmerised by its incredible therapeutic power and its gentle nature with minimal needle (De Qi) sensation. I love the embroidery-like patterns the needles make and the amazement on patients' faces as their pain leaves their body, often within minutes of the treatment commencing. The subtle nature of abdominal acupuncture ensures that the slightest adjustment of an abdominal needle can mean the difference between a successful treatment or not.

Abdominal acupuncture treatments often require fine tuning. Needles may have to be added, depths altered and Ahshi (painful) points penetrated until the desired result has been achieved. Within seconds an adjustment of a needle depth and/or location, by as little as a millimetre, can dramatically change the outcome of a treatment. This requires a certain amount of intuition, openness and fluidity to find the relevant acupuncture or Ahshi point in or around the area that one might expect.

I find this form of acupuncture intriguing, powerful and consistently reliable. This is especially true when compared to various other microforms such as scalp or ear, each of which I have seen to be very effective in their own right. Abdominal acupuncture, however, has a special magic and majesty that I feel deserved my dedicated devotion and time to master. Ever since my first class in this subject my appetite for abdominal acupuncture has been insatiable. I am still learning from each client and from every class I teach.

I was lucky enough to complete a number of internships with the above mentioned Dr. Han Yan over a period of 5 years. Dr. Han had trained with Professor Zhiyun Bo, the originator of abdominal acupuncture, since the late 1990s and she was one of his first students. Her clinic at Jiangzu Province Hospital is incredibly busy with 30 to 40 patients seen on any given morning.

While I studied with Dr. Han, abdominal acupuncture (Fu Zhen) was the therapy of choice in approximately 80-90% of cases. It was used either as a stand-alone treatment or in conjunction with other acupuncture modalities. An incredibly generous teacher, Dr. Han would always explain the rationale behind each treatment in a comprehensive manner. It was a privilege to have studied with such a considerate teacher and I hope that you will find that I have also been generous with the information provided in this book, giving you plenty of scope to play around with AA in your own clinical practice.

During the intervals when I was not studying in China, I took what I had learned and put it into practice in my Dublin-based clinic. Through experimentation I found that my results improved and over time I was confident enough to try various prescriptions to treat similar conditions. As a result I found what worked best and I have included these different potential approaches to treating all kinds of painful conditions.

I started teaching abdominal acupuncture to qualified acupuncturists and final year acupuncture students in 2011. Additionally, I completed a recognised *Train the Trainer, Level 6 (FETAC) course,* which gave me the tools to design, present and evaluate training courses using the most modern techniques so that all kinds of learning styles can be catered for. I designed and present these *Centreforce Abdominal Acupuncture* workshops myself. They are continually evolving and, as a result, I feel that I have found what I hope is a good system for teaching this form of acupuncture.

As a consequence of running each new course, my students have taught me a lot about how best to train people in the art of AA and the idea for this book evolved primarily from that. As well as really enjoying teaching my peers, the feedback I got from students who were getting great results using AA following each course made me want to share this system with a greater audience. Hence, a labour of love began with this project.

This book is a compilation of my experiences and is my interpretation of AA and how best to use it to get the effective and consistent results for all kinds of painful conditions. I hope that it will inspire you to become confident with using AA, so that you can become a master of this wonderful system of acupuncture.

Introduction

This book is intended for those with an interest in acupuncture. However, it is more specifically aimed at those who have studied acupuncture to a final year level and for those qualified acupuncturists who are looking for a more effective method of treating all kinds of painful muscular skeletal and sense organ problems. The book is a learning manual and thus it will teach you all relevant aspects of abdominal acupuncture necessary to treat a variety of conditions ranging from a slipped disc to frozen shoulder. It covers all sorts of sports injury and repetitive strains and deals with problems ranging from sciatic pain travelling down the leg to neuralgia in the fingers, the toes or anywhere in-between. After reading this book you will also be equipped to treat all kinds of sense organ problems such as painful eyes, ears or nasal congestion and various kinds of headache (See contents of chapter 7, *Prescriptions: What's the Point?* and chapter 8, *Abdominal Acupuncture Prescriptions for Frequently Seen Painful Conditions,* at the beginning of the book for more specifics.)

I have also detailed how to diagnose and treat conditions using the abdomen. I have provided much information on how you can formulate your own treatment plan (see chapter 9, *Putting it all Together*) for conditions that may not be covered in this book. You will gain confidence in reading and interpreting the abdomen, and you will get to know at a glance the familiar patterns that abdominal acupuncture points should present when treating various conditions.

As I noted already, in my first experience of AA I was both astonished and admiring of its effect. I hope that I can pass that same sense of awe onto you and that it will drive you to use this form as expertly as my tutor Dr. Han did.

Where to Find What You Want and How to Use This Book

As a learning manual, this book explains the mechanism and the theory behind abdominal acupuncture (See chapter 1, *Abdominal Acupuncture Theory*). It explains the function of the points (see chapter 4, *Points of the Abdomen*) used in this system and it offers two methods of point location (see chapter 3, *Abdominal Point Location...Get to the Point!*) as well as highlighting how to needle points (see chapter 6, *Abdominal Acupuncture Treatment Protocols*) when using abdominal acupuncture to treat various ailments. This book will teach you about the energetics of abdominal acupuncture (see chapter 2, *What Makes Abdominal So Phenomenal!*) and why it is more powerful than other so-called micro systems such as ear acupuncture.

You will also gain insight into diagnosis (see chapter 5, *Abdominal Diagnosis - Feel the Force*) through the abdomen and specifically how to locate and treat Ahshi points* in order to get the most powerful and effective results. You will learn a multitude of abdominal prescriptions (see chapter 7, *Prescriptions: What's the Point?* and chapter 8, *Abdominal Acupuncture Prescriptions for Frequently Seen Painful Conditions*) for all kinds of conditions that you are likely to encounter and these are supported with real case histories from my own clinic (all client names are changed to maintain client confidentiality). I recommend that you initially use this manual systematically and read it chapter-by-chapter.

*(Ahshi points may be a small node or nodule that is not necessarily very painful to touch, but because of the location, with respect to the anatomical area being reflected using the turtle hologram, will cure the painful part of the body being treated with AA.)

I hope that the book will be the start of a beautiful relationship between you and abdominal acupuncture. I encourage you to start using this amazing system after you finish reading. Follow the Centreforce system and you are sure to get good results. Please feel free to share your experiences with me and where necessary I will assist with difficult cases. **You can contact me through the website address at the end of this book.**

Abdominal Acupuncture: Some Special Features

Abdominal acupuncture (AA) is, in my opinion, one of the most exciting and innovative forms of acupuncture to evolve from China in decades, if not centuries. It was developed by Professor Zhiyun Bo and it has been used in China since 1991. It is also known as Bo's Method of Abdominal Acupuncture or (BMAA). I will refer to it as AA throughout this book.

Abdominal acupuncture is a micro-system of acupuncture and like other microforms, such as auricular acupuncture, all the organs and body parts are contained (reflected) within a small area. Abdominal acupuncture uses the area between Ren 12 (Zhongwan) and Ren 4 (Guanyuan) on the vertical line and Sp 15 (Daheng) as the outermost points on the horizontal lines. It uses points along the Ren, Kidney, Stomach and Spleen meridians primarily. There are also eight specific abdominal acupuncture (Ab) points that are unique to this system. All body parts and organs can be treated by needling within this small area.

AA works at three distinct levels. A blueprint of the turtle (see Fig I.1) is used to map the anatomical areas of the body at the most superficial (heaven) level, while the ancient Ba Gua (See chapter 1, *Abdominal Acupuncture Theory*) is used as a hologram to explain the relationship with the corresponding organs and viscera of the body at the deepest of the three levels known as earth.

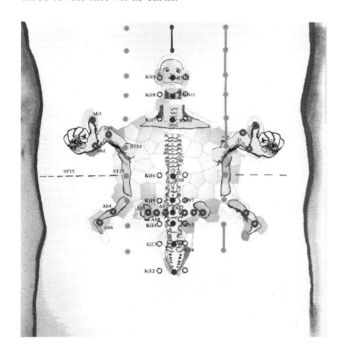

Fig I.1. Abdominal acupuncture chart of the turtle

Unlike other micro-systems AA is much more powerful as a result of its proximity with the Zang Fu organs and because it connects with all the meridians of the body (discussed later; see chapter 2, *What Makes Abdominal So Phenomenal!*).

As a therapy, it has become very popular in China because of its impressive results and its gentle nature (minimal needle sensation). The results are often achieved within moments of inserting the needle to the correct depth. It is very versatile and can treat all-over body pain in the one treatment, such as that seen with fibromyalgia (Bi Syndrome). It is particularly effective for treating paralysis due to stroke and is often used in preference to scalp acupuncture in the treatment of post-stroke sequelae. It is actually preferred as a treatment by the majority of my clients. Once it is mastered it is very easy to administer and to adapt for all kinds of painful conditions.

AA uses a concept familiar throughout TCM (Traditional Chinese Medicine) and acupuncture. That is, it uses three distinct levels, namely: heaven, humanity and earth. In traditional acupuncture these relevant depths are used in needling techniques such as tonification and reduction ('setting the mountain on fire' or 'penetrating heaven coolness'). These levels are also the three different depths used in pulse diagnosis.

The main focus of this book will be on using the heaven / superficial level to treat painful conditions of the body including the head, torso, upper and lower limbs. The heaven level is represented by the turtle/tortoise, an animal that has been highly revered in China for thousands of years (see chapter 1, *Abdominal Acupuncture Theory*).

There are a number of reasons why the turtle was chosen as a hologram of the human body (see chapter 1, *Abdominal Acupuncture Theory*). One such reason is that the plastron (underneath) of a turtle looks similar to a well-toned human abdomen, in other words, 'a six pack'. It's thus used in a similar way to how the image of an upside-down foetus is used to map the points on the ear in auricular acupuncture.

AA Main Points and Some of the Anatomical Significance

Since AA is bi-dimensional in nature points on the Ren can be used to treat the Du Mai and likewise points along the Kidney channel can be used to treat the Urinary Bladder meridian. Accurate point location is essential when using AA, and therapeutic results are dependent on correct location. For this reason I give a detailed description of different location methods in chapter 3. Therapeutic effect is also dependent on the depth of the needles, making it different from other forms of acupuncture. The depth of the needles ranges from very superficial 0.1 cun to deep at 1.5-2 cun, depending on the size of the client.

Main abdominal points (See Fig I.1 and I.2 abdominal acupuncture chart of the turtle).

- Ren 12 (Zhongwan) treats the head and is located specifically at the mouth;
- Ren 11 (Jianli) exerts its effect on the throat and neck and anatomically relates to the 1st cervical vertebra;
- Ren 10 (Xiawan) is located on a level with the 7th cervical vertebra;
- Ren 9 (Shuifen) is equivalent to the 7th thoracic vertebra;
- Ren 6 (Qihai) coincides with the 1st lumbar vertebra;
- Ren 4 (Guanyuan) is the tail of the turtle and relates to the 4th or 5th lumbar vertebra;

- St 25 (Tianshu) treats the mid back area;
- Sp 15 (Daheng) is the outer boundary of the turtle;
- St 24 (Huaroumen) corresponds with the shoulder. The elbow is found 0.5 cun superior and lateral to this while the wrist is found 0.5 cun inferior and lateral to the elbow. This gives the shape of an inverted V;
- St 26 (Wailing) corresponds with the hip point. The knee is found 0.5 cun inferior and lateral to the hip point, and the ankle point is on a line 0.5 cun lateral and inferior to the knee point. Hip, knee and ankle should look like a backslash \.

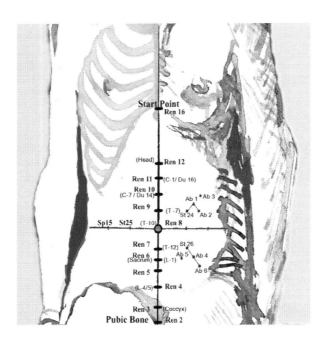

Fig I.2. Simplified abdominal acupuncture chart of the turtle

Standard Uses in China

Since its introduction in 1991 abdominal acupuncture has gained in popularity as a treatment form. It has been readily accepted because the patient outcome is so good and as a result of the almost painless nature of the needle sensation. In 2007 abdominal acupuncture was recognised as a professional subcommittee under the *China Acupuncture and Moxibustion Association*. Today abdominal acupuncture is recognised in the treatment of all kinds of muscular–skeletal pain including stiff neck, cervical vertebra problems, frozen shoulder and scapular-humeral periarteritis, arthritis, cervical, dorsum and lumbar spondylopathy, lumbar pain with sciatica, tennis elbow, tendonitis, wrist problems such as carpal tunnel, hip, knee and ankle problems, and orthopaedic problems. It also treats many cerebro–vascular conditions including hemiplegia and hypertension, Parkinson's disease and other neurological conditions (D'Alberto, A. and Kim, E. 2005).

Additionally, abdominal acupuncture treats all manner of digestive conditions including diabetes and diabetic neuritis, gynaecological and disturbances of the nervous system including anxiety, insomnia and depression. You will also find that it is an effective treatment for respiratory and coronary heart disease.

Between 1999 and 2007, 214 articles have been published on abdominal acupuncture in China, including 96 clinical trials, of which 62 used comparative treatment for control groups. Of the 74 musculoskeletal diseases studied, 30 were for cervical spondylosis with nerve root compression. Of those, 22 used comparative treatment control groups.

Efficacy was more than 90%. Among the 22 studies, a multi-site study was conducted in 2005 at three hospitals in which 300 subjects were randomised into abdominal acupuncture and traction therapy treatment groups. Traction therapy was found to 'improve local Blood circulation and relieve symptoms, but lacked stable, long term curative effects which led to frequent relapses,' while the cure rate with abdominal acupuncture reached 91.5% (complete remission within ten treatments and no return for three months) and an efficacy rate of 98% (Ryan, P. 2011).

A study comparing the effectiveness of abdominal acupuncture with electro acupuncture in the treatment of 98 cases of prolapsed intervertebral disc revealed the following results (see Table I.1):

Abdominal Acupuncture	Electro Acupuncture
40% Completely effective	29.1% Completely effective
48% Significantly effective	41.7% Significantly effective
12% Slightly effective	20.8% Slightly effective
0% No effect	9.3% No effect

Table I.1 Comparison of electro and abdominal acupuncture. (Guo. F, et al, 2003)

Advantages of Abdominal Acupuncture

✓ Less needle sensation, therefore, less painful and clients generally prefer it. Needles are usually of a low gauge 0.16-0.25 mm and are therefore less noticeable for the client;

✓ AA uses shallow needling so less risk of injury. Therefore when using abdominal acupuncture to treat knee problems there is no risk of causing an infection whereas using knee eye points such as St 35 (Dubi) have a higher risk of causing an infection;

✓ Like other microforms of acupuncture, AA avoids the necessity to treat injuries where there might be swelling or bandages preventing local access;

✓ Usually abdominal acupuncture achieves better efficacy than other microforms;

✓ It is especially good for painful and chronic conditions. Due to the Biao-Li relationship and the location of the Zang Fu organs on the abdomen results can be superior to those achieved by needling distal points. This can prove less effective when there are nodes or blockages along the pathways that prevent the transmission of stimulation getting to the organs and viscera; (Ryan. P. 2009);

✓ It is good for those with a weak constitution, including the elderly and/or immuno–compromised clients;

✓ Abdominal acupuncture is easier to administer to oneself and can treat various conditions without having to stretch to needle distal points. (I have used it on many occasions to fix my back!);

✓ It can treat a large number of problems at once - Conditions such as fibromyalgia, which can cause pain at all joints of the limbs as well as different areas of the back can be addressed in one abdominal acupuncture treatment (see chapter 8, case history, 'Accident Prone Anita');

✓ It gives rapid results. When emphasised by the pain scale of 1-10 a reduction to a score of 2-3 will amaze your clients and this will encourage them to talk about the experience and refer more patients to you;

✓ Energetically powerful results can take 24-48 hours to become evident. Clients will often notice improvements in their condition over this period;

✓ There is less likelihood of abdominal acupuncture aggravating painful conditions in the way that local points can;

✓ AA is unlikely to cause a client to faint, unlike some stronger acupuncture points such as Master Tung point Ling Gu. (see case history, 'Not for the Faint Hearted (Master Tung points for Backache)' below;

✓ You can charge more for abdominal acupuncture. (I charge 10% more for AA in my practice);

✓ There are only a few practitioners using abdominal acupuncture, which will give you an advantage over your competitors;

✓ I find that AA often gives more profound, diverse and comprehensive side benefits than traditional acupuncture gives. (See 'New Lease of Life' below).

CASE STUDY: Not for the Faint Hearted (Master Tung points for Backache)

Brian, a busy businessman, came for acupuncture on advice from his sister after he sprained his back playing tennis. He had never had acupuncture and was in a lot of pain with severely restricted movement on his right side when he arrived. I was busy but I decided to fit him in as he was in agony.

His problem was primarily related to the foot Shao Yang (GB) and the foot Tai Yang (UB) meridians. Most of his pain was at GB 30 (Huantiao) and radiated down his right leg to UB 40 (Weizhong).

Due to time constraints he was treated with a combination of traditional and Master Tung acupuncture. Using channel palpation techniques (Dr. Wang Ju Yi), it was decided to use UB 63 (Jinmen) GB 30 (Huantiao) UB 40 (Weizhong) all on the right and Ling Gu on the left.

The needles were left for 20 minutes and, after removing all the needles except Ling Gu, I decided to stimulate this powerful hand point while Brian moved his lower back. After stimulating Ling Gu for a minute Brian's complexion turned ashen and he became faint. He was laid out on the plinth, and the needle was removed and Du 26 (Renzhong) was massaged to help resuscitate him.

Brian later acknowledged that he was squeamish about needles and would faint when having blood taken. He recovered well and was happy with the result that had improved his condition by seventy per cent. He was informed that future sessions would use less intensive procedures, mainly abdominal acupuncture.

On his next visit Brian's movement was much improved but he still had pain at GB 30 (Huantiao) and UB 40 (Weizhong) and his movement, although it was better, would not allow him to play his much-loved tennis. The treatment was kept minimal the points used were Ren 6 (Qihai) Ren 4 (Guanyuan) Ab 7 (Qipang) on the left, St 26 (Wailing) bilaterally and Ab 4 (knee pt) on the right. Ahshi points were noticed at both right St 26 (Wailing) and Ab 4 which reflected the pain at GB 30 (Huantiao) and UB 40 (Weizhong) respectively. Following needling of these Ahshi points pain levels were checked and both areas showed a marked reduction in pain (see Fig I.3). Brian found the abdominal treatment much gentler and, having had reservations about returning, he was once again committed to continuing with acupuncture.

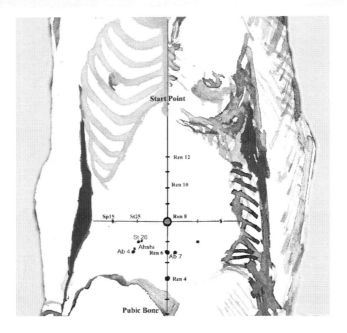

Fig I.3. Prescription used for case history 'Not for the Faint Hearted'

CASE STUDY: A New Lease of Life

A 55-year-old new client was suffering from debilitating, deafening (low pitched) tinnitus, rock-bottom energy and a generally low mood. However, he commented after his first ever AA treatment that he felt as if he were seventeen years old again. Following the treatment he felt so invigorated, he told me that he wanted to do a hundred-metre sprint. I told him to enjoy his new lease of life and to preserve his vigour. His original diagnosis was one of Liver and Kidney Yin Vacuity. He had signs of Spleen Qi and Yang Deficiency and was frequently tired. He worked different shifts and his symptoms were aggravated after nights of intense, concentrated twelve hour periods of computer work.

On his second visit he was happy that the tinnitus was gone for four days until he returned to night work. Once again he felt invigorated as never before with traditional acupuncture. The pain he suffered in his right arm as a result of cervical vertebrae (C-5) surgery disappeared after the first treatment. He informed me that his energy, sleep, mood, focus and outlook on life were all much better and that although the tinnitus had returned he could tolerate it as he felt so good and so vibrant!

While he had a good experience and great results with traditional acupuncture years previously, he described the results from AA as on a totally different plane.

Disadvantages

✓ It is easier to bruise due to the large number of Blood vessels supplying the area. Bruises tend to be colourful not painful. Always advise clients if they bleed that they will get a bruise that might be present for 7-10 days. (Arnica cream will clear up the haematoma quickly);

✓ Abdominal acupuncture can take longer to administer if there are a lot of symptoms to be treated.

Abdominal Acupuncture Spreads from China throughout the World

As abdominal acupuncture gains momentum its popularity has spread beyond Asia. It is used throughout Europe, Australia and America. However, this is the first book on the topic to be published in English. Although AA is moving across the continents it is still relatively new and is currently only used by a minority of practitioners. So you should you use it; it will give you an edge over your competition.

I recommend that as soon as you have completed this book you start to apply all that you have learned. Abdominal acupuncture is very versatile and, once practiced, it is easy to adapt to individual cases. Results are rapid and, therefore, confidence grows as a result. Use this book as your guide and learn the main anatomical regions of the body as represented by the turtle hologram. Remember to be fluid, people are different and locations of points can be slightly different too. Be open and listen to your intuition. Follow this advice and you will soon have mastered the art of abdominal acupuncture.

Chapter 1: Abdominal Acupuncture Theory

Learning Objectives

I will start the first chapter of this book by teaching you how Prof. Bo discovered AA and how he developed this system. We will look at the special significance of the point Ren 8 (Shenque) concerning the Abdominal Meridian System (AMS) as proposed by Prof. Bo. We will also look at the anatomy of the umbilicus to understand its importance concerning the congenital and acquired (pre- and postnatal) Abdominal Meridian Systems (AMS). You will learn about the different levels of the abdomen, namely heaven, humanity, and earth, and how they are used to treat the body at different levels. We will also explore the ancient history behind the Ba Gua theory and the reason the turtle acts as a hologram for the human anatomical regions.

General Considerations

The first AA weekend course I studied in China (with someone other than Dr. Han Yan) was difficult to understand, partly because of the Pigeon English but also due to the amount of theory that was approximately 85% of the fourteen hours! When I studied with Dr. Han in the busy hospital, she explained cases when we had time between patients. Training with Dr. Han was 90% practical and the rest was discussion and theory.

In this book I'm trying to cater for all levels and, therefore, need to balance theory with some practical elements. I hope I have achieved this successfully! All you need to understand from this chapter is the four core points of the AMS. The rest is an attempt to show that this all goes back to the ancient teachings and that what was true then remains true now. This is a concept that amazes and excites me. It gives me the utmost admiration for ancient Chinese culture that proves again and again that it is timeless. It is relevant to all kinds of modern scientific disciplines and has a depth that is both fascinating and unfathomable to me.

Abdominal Acupuncture Genesis through Sciatica

Abdominal acupuncture was conceived by Prof. Zhiyun Bo in 1972. The professor had a client with a particularly difficult case of sciatica that had not responded to any western techniques or other form of acupuncture including ear, scalp and traditional acupuncture methods. Puzzled but undaunted he looked to other possible solutions to treat his patient.

The ancient Chinese concept of Biao (external) and Li (internal) is an ideology that uses parallelism and dualism and dates back to between the 5th and 2nd century BC. These parallel and dualistic ideas of Biao-Li are found in various branches of Chinese literature, poetry, art, cosmology and traditional Chinese medicine (TCM). The ancient turtle shell gave rise to this Biao–Li idea. Observation indicated that the turtle has two possibilities -the upper shell represents heaven while the underneath represents the earth. It is, in effect, a microcosm of the world we live in (Peluffo, E. 2014, pp. 270-276).

These philosophical and scientific concepts gave rise to the theory of Yin-Yang (Parallelism paradigm, Heaven: Man used in TCM) and five phases/elements, amongst others. The parallel pairings are also seen with the manner in which the Zang Fu organs were combined, i.e. Yin (internal) Lung is paired with its Yang (external) Large Intestine, (see Table 1.1, below), which were discussed in detail in the ancient writings of Su Wen.

Internal, Yin, Zang Organ	External, Yang, Fu Organ
Lung	Large Intestine
Spleen	Stomach
Heart	Small Intestine
Kidney	Urinary Bladder
Liver	Gall Bladder
Pericardium	San Jiao / Triple Burner

Table 1.1. The parallel pairings of the Zang Fu organs/meridians

From a Yin-Yang, and channel pairing perspective it follows that the Ren Mai (Yin) can treat the Du Mai (Yang) just as the Kidney can treat the Urinary Bladder through the Biao-Li connection (see Table 1.1).

Considering these concepts, Professor Bo decided to treat the case of sciatica by using the points Ren 6 (Qihai) and Ren 4 (Guanyuan). The results were powerful and rapid. The pain was cured within five minutes of inserting the needles and for the first time Prof. Bo's patient's sciatic pain was gone. In fact, so successful was this path that the professor had taken, his patient's sciatica was cured completely after just one treatment (D'Alberto, A. and Kim, E. 2005). Prof. Bo continued to use this prescription to treat other similar cases with the same impressive results. Based on the above principles and the fact that Ren 6 (Qihai) is on a line equivalent to the first lumbar vertebra (L-1) and Ren 4 (Guanyuan) is on a line with L-4 or L-5, Professor Bo realised that there was much potential in using the abdomen to treat all kinds of pain and other disharmonies. Therein began a lifetime of research and development of abdominal acupuncture.

Development of the Abdominal Acupuncture System

After achieving such good results, Professor Bo set to work researching and developing the abdominal meridian system (AMS) theory upon which abdominal acupuncture is based. After 20 years he was ready to introduce it. In 1991 Bo's Method of Abdominal Acupuncture (B. M. A. A.) won the acupuncture and Tui-na massage competition organised by the Shangxi regional Ministry of Health (Ryan, P. 2009).

Ancient History behind Abdominal Acupuncture

Throughout the ages and different traditions the abdomen has played a pivotal role in health and medical fields. In ancient disciplines such as Tai Chi Chuan, Qi Gong and medical massage such as Qi Nei Zang the abdomen is of paramount importance. Japanese therapies such as Acupuncture, Shiatsu and Kampo herbal therapy continued to use the abdomen for both diagnosis and treatment. In China this skill was mainly forgotten, due primarily to taboos of indecency. In Tai Chi Chuan, the umbilicus Ren 8 (Shenque) is the centre of the Tai Qi symbol (Fig 1.1).

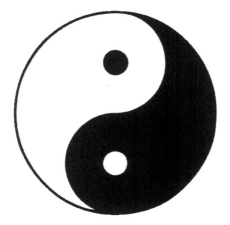

Fig 1.1. Yin -Yang or Tai Qi symbol

The Abdominal Meridian System (AMS)

There are four main points to the AMS theory as stated by Prof. Bo in his paper, *The Importance of the Acupoint Shenque in the Study of Abdominal Acupuncture.*

1. Ren 8 (Shenque) at the embryological stage is the regulator of all macroscopic systems of the body;
2. Ren 8 (Shenque) is the mother of all the meridian systems of the body;
3. The Shenque system is responsible for the Qi communication between the meridians, the auto regulation of the Blood vessels and therefore of Blood circulation;

4. It also acts as the core centre of the meridian system.

Professor Bo postulated that the body has two abdominal meridian systems. These both originate from the umbilicus, i.e. the point Ren 8 (Shenque). These two AMS's modulate the movement of Qi and Blood throughout the body at different stages of development. The AMS is the source or 'mother', from which all the meridian regulatory systems develop. The standard primary (Jing Luo) meridian system only develops after the baby's own Zang Fu organs are functioning and producing post-heaven Qi.

The Pre-Heaven or Congenital Abdominal Meridian System (AMS)

The congenital or first abdominal meridian system (AMS) is formed during conception and develops throughout the pregnancy until birth. It originates from the umbilicus, Ren 8 (Shenque), which is the central point of the abdomen and it is where all cell division radiates from after the sperm and ovum unite to form a zygote and blastocyst.

This congenital AMS provides all the nutritional and other requirements of the developing baby from the mother's placenta via the umbilical cord. It forms a circulatory system that facilitates the movement of these nutrients from the umbilicus to all parts of the growing foetus. In this way the congenital (first) or prenatal AMS regulates all Qi and Blood throughout the whole body of the developing baby until birth.

As soon as the baby is born it takes its first breath. From this moment onwards it gets all nutrients and air from an external source (post-heaven Qi). The umbilical cord is cut and it forms a scar, i.e. the belly button which is the location of Ren 8 (Shenque). The umbilicus undergoes huge change over the next few days and is no longer the main source of nutrients. However the first AMS still retains a function as a regulator of Qi and Blood. This function is maintained throughout the rest of one's life. This explains the therapeutic effect of abdominal acupuncture at the heaven level.

The Second / Post-Heaven (Natal) or Acquired AMS

As the umbilicus closes it develops into nerve tissues and forms a second circulatory system, i.e. the second, postnatal or acquired AMS. At this stage the new role of the second AMS takes over. As the baby matures and the Zang Fu organs grow the baby's own Jing Lou meridian system begins to develop.

Both the pre- (first) and post-heaven (second) AMS communicate via the middle level standard Jing Lou meridian system so that they can regulate all parts and organs of the body.

It can be seen that the (Shenque) Ren 8 system acts as a modulator of Qi and Blood from the very conception of the baby. It is also the central point of the three-tiered abdominal system. This explains why the depth of the needles is so crucial when using abdominal acupuncture.

The Physiological Make-Up of the Umbilicus and its Significance to AA

The umbilicus is made up of (Fig 1.2). (Yang C. 2012, pp 185-188):

- A yolk sac stalk that later goes on to make up the intestines;
- Allantois which later becomes the Urinary Bladder;
- Urachus afterbirth that becomes fibres and connective tissue;
- Two arteries that supply Blood, Qi, oxygen and nutrients to the developing foetus;
- One vein which carries carbon dioxide and waste materials from the foetus.

From this physiological view of the umbilicus it should be apparent that the point Ren 8 (Shenque) is indeed the foundation of the genesis of human development.

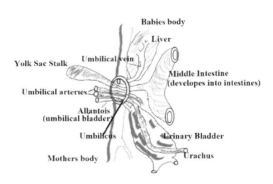

Fig 1.2. The structure of the umbilicus during embryogenesis

The Three Layers of the Abdomen in AA

"…It is said that the energy of the heaven takes charge of the region above the centre of the universe and that the energy of the earth takes charge of the region below the centre of the universe; the energy of man is guided by the region in which communication of energy takes place and from which the origin of everything is derived" (Lu H C, 1978, p 441).

- **Heaven / superficial level** this is the prenatal or congenital (first) AMS formed during the development of the embryo. This level lies just under the skin and treats all kinds of pain in all regions including head (and sense organs), torso, upper and lower limbs. It also treats acute disorders (meridian and collateral disorders). It is represented by a hologram of the turtle/tortoise (see Fig 1.3) and it contains Bo's new abdominal points (Ab 1-8). It is the most frequently used layer and is the main focus of this book.
- **Humanity / middle level** is found in the fat layer and it connects the internal and external. It forms a connection between the congenital and the acquired AMS. It is based on the Jing Lou theory and uses standard primary and extraordinary meridians to treat the body.
- **Earth / deep level** is located in the muscle layer on the acquired (postnatal/second) AMS. It treats the Zang Fu organs and viscera and chronic conditions it is represented by the Ba Gua /8 trigrams (see Fig 1.4).

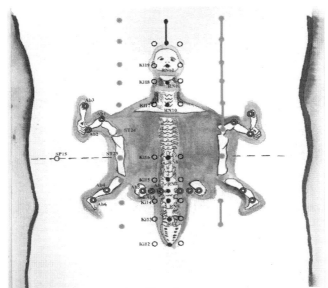

Fig 1.3. Abdominal acupuncture chart of the turtle

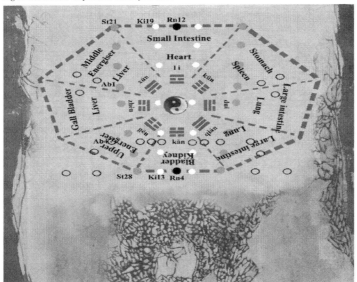

Fig 1.4. Abdominal acupuncture Ba Gua chart

Ancient Thinking by Numbers

Ancient Chinese numerology, particularly the cosmic boxes or magic squares, which date back over 2000 years B.C. have been used to explain all manner of phenomenon. Abdominal acupuncture theory also uses the ancient magic number boxes of the He Tou (Fig 1.5) and the Lou Shu (Fig 1.4) which are said to predate Yin-Yang, 5 elements (or 5 phases), and many other traditional Chinese medicine (TCM) theories (Yang-Li, 1998, p.6).

2	7	4
3	5	9
8	1	6

Fig 1.5. The He Tou magic square

Both the He Tu and the Lou Shu cosmic boxes were ruminated upon by many of the great masters over time. From their analysis came various new theories, including the Ba Gua, which were discussed at length in such masterpieces as the Ling Shu and the I Ching (Yi Ching).

4	9	2
3	5	7
8	1	6

From these magic number boxes the early and later heaven Ba Gua formations arose. The later heaven Ba Gua is used to formulate the abdominal Ba Gua hologram (see Fig 1.4).

Fig 1.6. The Lou Shu magic square

Wisdom Springs from the Ancient Tortoise

The Lou Shu turtle writing was found by the great ruler Yu on the back of a divine tortoise that came out of the Lou River. The turtle is three-dimensional and has the magic square on its shell (fig 1.7), which consists of 3 rows of 3 squares. Any combination of 3 in a row will add up to 15 and any 3 numbers in a line of the magic square will total 15.

Wood	Fire	Earth
4	9	2
Xun (Wind)	Li (Fire)	Kun (Earth)
Liver	Ht / SI	Sp / St
(Middle		
Burner)		
Wood	Earth	Metal
3	5	7
Zhen	Kun	Dui (Lake)
(Thunder)	Primordial	Lung / LI
Liv / GB	Qi	(lower Burner)
Earth	Water	Metal
8	1	6
Gen	Kan	Qian
(Mountain)	(Water)	(heaven)
Upper Burner	Kid / UB	Lung / LI

Fig 1.7. The Lou Shu Magic Square with the 5 phases and the later heaven Ba Gua reflecting the relevant organ treated by each Gua

The dome of the shell depicts heaven; the body is humanity and the plastron is earth. The number sequence through the turtle is 9-5-1 (Li, no. 9) Fire, (Kun no. 5) earth and (Kan no. 1) water. The water element is where we all originate from and an imaginary womb or navel is found here (Tuvla, S. 2012).

As early as the 6th century there are references found in the 'Classic of nine halls (palaces) calculation of the Yellow Emperor'. Chen Luan, an influential Taoist of the time, discussed how the turtle Lou Shu number chart represents the human body:

- 2 and 4 make shoulders;
- 6 and 8 make feet;
- 3 is at the left, 7 is at the right;
- 9 is worn in the head;
- 1 is underfoot;
- 5 dwells in the centre.

Professor Zhiyun Bo further developed the concept of the turtle as a blueprint by adding his own new abdominal points (Ab points, see Fig 1.4 above). He completed the picture with Ab 1 and 2 representing the elbow and wrist in the same shape of a turtle's front fins, i.e. an inverted V shape. Ab 4 represents the knee and Ab 6 is the ankle. These are in a diagonal line like a backslash \ as are the turtle's back fins.

From Cosmic Number Boxes to the Ba Gua

These two early cosmic number diagrams (the He Tu and the Lou Shu) gave rise to two different Ba Gua (8 trigram) formations in the Yijing or I Ching ('Book of Changes'). Named after their inventors they became known as the Fu Xi and King Wen 8 trigram (8 Gua or Bagua) formations. They are used to explain many theories in Chinese medicine, and indeed many aspects of modern science, from the theory of relativity to the 64 possible codons that make up DNA in genetics (L. Yang, 2008, p.37). The *Collections of Einstein* contains this statement: 'It is a miracle that all these discoveries had already been made (in China)', acknowledging that the Bagua can be used to explain many complex theories that Einstein developed!

These two formations are similar. However in the later heaven Ba Gua, as developed by King Wen, the Li trigram denoting the fire element is no.9 and takes place at the top south (Yang position), while the Kǎn trigram with the lowest no.1 Yin position is at the bottom or north of the circular format, representing the water element. This is the format that is used to represent the deep level (earth) in abdominal acupuncture (see Figs 1.4 and 1.7).

The Ba Gua is a logical system that is credited as being the first mathematical binary system (1:0, used in computers) (Dr. Richard Tan, 2013, personal communication). The Ba Gua / 8 trigrams uses a series of lines (Yao) to denote the energetic transformative state of Qi. A broken line - - indicates Yin while, an unbroken line - depicts Yang energy. The trigrams have three lines (Yao), which give details of the various transformative states of Qi in all kinds of natural cycles, e.g. hourly, daily, seasonal, menstrual cycles etc. The number three once again is used as it is frequently found in Chinese medical systems:

- 1 gives life to 2: Yin, Yang
- 2 gives life to 3: Tai Chi or Ba Gua (8 trigrams)
- 3 or Tai Chi gives life to all things.

Each Yao is very important as it can represent a multitude of things including Shen, Qi and Jing or heaven, humanity and earth at different stages or cycles of time.

Together the nine palaces, the He Tu, and Lou Shu variations in cosmic digital diagrams and the early and later Ba Gua can all be used to explain a myriad of theories. These include abdominal acupuncture, Chinese philosophy, astrology, Feng Shui, Yin-Yang, 5 elements, Zang Fu and many more Chinese medicine concepts, mirror imaging and acupuncture balancing techniques, as well as martial arts and military strategy.

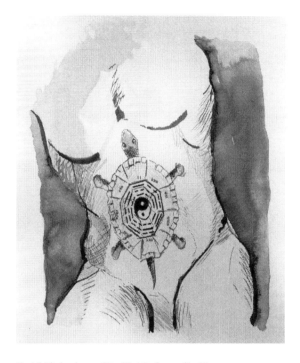

Fig 1.8. The late heaven (King Wen) Ba Gua used in AA

The Abdominal Ba Gua

The late heaven (King Wen) format of the Ba Gua is used as a hologram in abdominal acupuncture at the third and deepest level, which is referred to as the earth level (see Figs 1.4 and 1.8). The trigram Li in the south is the fire element and treats the Heart and its paired Yang organ, the Small

Intestine (SI). These organs can be treated by needling this area to a depth of between 1.00-1.5 or in larger subjects 2.00cun. Moving in a clockwise direction (Fig 1.4, 1.7 and 1.8) the trigram Kūn (earth in the five elements/phases) is the Spleen and Stomach area and, for this reason, the elbow point (Ab 1) on the patients left is used to treat Excess and/or Deficient conditions of the Spleen. Continuing around the trigram of Dui (lake) is the metal element, the area of the Lungs and Large Intestine (LI). This trigram houses St 25 (Tianshu) which is the front Mu of the LI and is often used to clear Heat from all areas. St 25 (Tianshu) is also used to treat asthma and other Lung conditions such as a cough. The Qian (heaven) trigram also treats Lung and LI conditions. The trigram of Kǎn, water is situated at the north directly opposite the fire in the south, and it represents the water organs of the Kidney and Urinary Bladder. This area contains two of the most powerful Kidney tonifying points, Ren 6 (Qihai) and Ren 4 (Guanyuan). Continuing around the trigram Gen (mountain) treats conditions of the upper Burner. Zhen (Thunder) is on the patient's right and it represents the Gallbladder and Liver. The trigram of Xun (Wind) is the final segment and it represents the element of wood and therefore treats the Liver and the middle Burner. The elbow point (Ab 1) in this segment is used to treat conditions related to Liver Qi Stagnation.

Why Use a Hologram of the Turtle / Tortoise?

- The divine tortoise / the miraculous turtle has been highly revered in Chinese mythology for millennia;
- The plastron of the turtle resembles the abdomen of humans (more so if you have a well-defined abdomen);

- The divine tortoise gave the inspiration for the concept of Biao-Li, which led to Yin-Yang, 5 elements (Wu Xi) and other very important fundamental philosophies of TCM, Feng Shui, cosmology and much more;
- The miraculous turtle is said to have carried the Lou Shu magic square on its shell. This number square led to the development of the later heaven format of the Ba Gua which is used in AA;
- The area of the Dantian is also known as the Great Sea or Da Hai, where the 'Spirit Turtle' resides.

Summary of Topics Covered in this Chapter

1. The four main points to the AMS theory as stated by Prof. Zhiyun Bo
2. An understanding of the three layers of the abdomen heaven, humanity and earth
3. How each level is represented and what each layer treats
4. The origins and relevance of the abdominal Ba Gua
5. Why the turtle/tortoise is the blueprint at the heaven/superficial level.

Chapter 2: What Makes Abdominal So Phenomenal!

Learning Objectives

In this chapter you will learn about the special significance of the abdomen. This will be addressed from a number of important factors, including historical relevance Yuan Qi and the San Jiao / Triple Burner (I use these terms interchangeably as they are referred to by both descriptions in various quotes), the proximity of the Zang Fu organs and the twelve regular and the extraordinary meridians. I also present more recent (conventional/Western) scientific evidence to support the potential power and mechanisms of abdominal acupuncture. .

General Considerations

As I mentioned in the preface, my first encounter with AA 'blew me away'. I observed a patient in Dr. Han Yan's clinic become completely free of severe frozen shoulder pain within minutes. This was a transformative moment for me. I was excited and delighted to see the look of joy and amazement on the lady's face as she recovered full mobility of her shoulder in a completely pain-free manner. With many of my treatments and Centreforce demonstrations of AA, I get that same 'internal cartwheel moment' when AA cures peoples' pain rapidly.

I hope that I can somehow give you, the reader, the same sense of wonderment regarding AA and that it will drive you to become an expert, with an assurance that AA will be miraculous in your hands also.

I have always found AA both intriguing and reliable. For these reasons I tried to be as comprehensive with my research as possible. I have experienced the power of AA on all kinds of practical levels, but articles on the subject are limited. Thus, I have given a lot of time to present evidence in support of the potential mechanisms of AA in this book. I find it all incredible and yet obvious that the modern scientific evidence consolidates the ancient and modern Chinese TCM scientific theory.

Special Significance of the Abdomen throughout the Ages in TCM

The abdomen is energetically very important in Chinese medicine and has been written about in many of the ancient classic books such as the *Neijing*, the earliest surviving work on Chinese medicine. The abdomen includes the area known as the 'Dantian', field of cinnabar or 'field of elixir', i.e. the abdomen is recognised as our 'energy centre'. These names reflect the importance and great power attached to the abdomen. Many of the abdominal acupuncture point names also emphasise the celestial or heavenly power of the area surrounding the umbilicus:

- Ren 8 (Shenque) means 'Spirit Gate' and it is said to be entrance and exit point of the shen. (Ellis, A et Al, 1998);
- St 25 (Tianshu) translates as 'Heavens / Heavenly Pivot';
- St 23 (Taiyi) is the 'Supreme Unity';

- Ren 3 (Zhongji) is the 'Central Pole' (Tuvla, S. 2008).

The area of the lower Dantian, including the points Ren 6 (Qihai) and Ren 4 (Guanyuan), is said to be the seat of the body's Yuan (source) Qi and Jing (Essence). This area is where our life force emanates from and is a focal point in most forms of meditation, Qi Gong, Tai Chi and other such esoteric and martial arts practices. This is where our centre of gravity lies.

"The Kidney is the gate of Qi generation. It emerges from and governs (the area) below the umbilicus, and it is divided into 3 forks surging upward through the umbilicus via the celestial pivot (St25 Tianshu) ascending to reach the chest centre Ren 17 (Shangzhong) beside both breasts. This is where the primal Qi is tied in," (Chace, C. & Shima, M., 2010, p. 27).

The next quote, from the Ching Dynasty physician Chang Chin-Chiou, emphasises the importance of the navel in his commentary on the *Yellow Emperor's Classic of Internal Medicine* (Reid, D.P. p146, 2001):

"Man is born attached at the navel to an umbilical cord, and the navel is connected to the lower elixir field, which is the Sea of Energy. Thus, the navel forms the Gate of Life. The foetus receives life through the opening of this Gate, and the infant enters this world by its closing. Therefore, in its capacity as a spring of living energy, this area is the source of a man's energy, this area is the source of a man's well-being and his discomfort, his strength and his weakness. When the energy here is strong, the whole system is strong. When it is weak, the whole system grows weak."

The navel is where Fire and Water meet, where Yin and Yang reside. It is the sea of essence and energy, the door of life and death."

The above quotes and terms for the area surrounding Ren 8 (Shenque) highlight the importance of the area and give Professor Bo's AMS theory a more valid foundation.

The Vicinity of the Zang Fu Organs to the Abdomen

All the Zang Fu organs reside in this area and can be accessed either directly or through the AMS connection.

The abdomen contains all the organs of the middle and lower Jiao. Although the Heart and Lungs are located in the upper Jiao/Burner they are connected with the abdomen via their Zang Fu coupled organs, namely the Large Intestine and the Small Intestine. The Heart in the chest is nourished by the Stomach and Spleen and has an internal/external relationship with the Small Intestine. The Lung channel begins in the middle Burner and connects with the Large Intestine. The Stomach and Spleen are located in the middle Burner. (Lore, R. 2011). The Gallbladder is also located in the middle Burner. The Kidneys, Liver and Urinary Bladder are found in the lower Burner. The Pericardium is the protective envelope surrounding the Heart and is thus located in the upper Burner. As its Zang Fu organ pair is the Triple Burner (TB), it can be accessed via the Triple Burner and, therefore, the abdomen. The Triple Burner combines all three areas of the chest, middle and lower abdominal regions and thus can be accessed easily using abdominal acupuncture (see below for more details on the TB).

Since all the Zang Fu organs are accessible through the abdomen, this gives abdominal acupuncture extra potency when compared to some other so-called microforms of acupuncture such as ear or scalp acupuncture. Abdominal acupuncture is now favoured in many Chinese hospitals over scalp acupuncture in the treatment of hemiplegia due to stroke.

The Abdomen's Special Relationship with the San Jiao / Triple Burner

A look at the all illusive and divisive (both physically and intellectually) organ that is said to have no form, though certainly has plenty of function, will help to illuminate the incredible power of the abdominal area.

The Triple Burner not only comprises the upper, middle and lower Burner and all the Zang Fu organs contained within, it also encompasses all passageways within the body. This allows for such far-reaching communication between organs via the network of passageways which includes extracellular and interstitial fluids.

Through this network Qi transformation occurs at a cellular level. This is as a result of the TB providing the pathway and the spark for the Yuan (source) Qi from the gate of vitality (Kidneys) to move throughout the body. At a cellular level it carries prenatal, Yuan and postnatal (Ying) nutrient Qi for all the body's metabolic processes.

It also regulates communication between all organs and cells of the body by facilitating the flow of cellular messengers' hormones and enzymes around the body, while at the same time removing all wastes from the cells through the elaborate passageways (Wang, J. & Robertson, J. 2008).

Its formless nature that utilises every space in the body including all types of connective tissue, such as facia, nerves and the spaces between joints and, therefore, includes synovial fluid. This fact accounts for the TB's use in treating joint problems.

In fact the TB can be given credit for holding the body in shape and sectioning off different organs and areas using facia. Facia is the connective tissue that holds everything together. It holds muscle to organs, to bone, nerves and skin. It has particular electrical properties in that it can produce and conduct electricity, it is a semiconductor. These properties make facia ideal for performing the function of acupuncture points. Facia explains acupuncture theory and the very nature of meridians (Jing) and collaterals (Luo) which connect all aspects of the body (Keown, D., 2014, pp. 12-15, loc 260-297, kindle format).

As a result of its diverse meanderings, complex nature and functions, the TB can be used to treat a variety of musculoskeletal, digestive, Zang Fu, Qi, Essence and Blood problems.

The abdomen houses the middle and the lower Burners. Of the three Burner's the abdominal area also has access to the upper Burner by its connection with the Lung and Large Intestine and the Heart and Small Intestine as discussed earlier. This connection with the Triple Burner and the importance of the points listed below, help to give further understanding to the potential power of the abdomen and, therefore, AA.

- Ren-12 Zhongwan harmonises the middle Burner and is a meeting point of the TB;

- Ren 9 (Shuifen) gives access to the middle Burner to stimulate the descending of Stomach-Qi, the transportation and transformation (Yun Hua) by the Spleen and the rotting and ripening by the Stomach (Maciocia, G. 2005, pp.211-212). It also regulates the water passages;
- Ren 7 (Yin Jiao) treats the lower Burner and helps its function of separating the clear and turbid from food and fluids;
- Ren 5 (Shimen) also accesses the lower Burner and the TB as a whole due to the fact that it is the front mu point of the TB;
- St 25 (Tianshu) addresses the middle Burner, which is the warm cauldron where the transformation of food and fluids movement of Qi is neither up nor down. Instead, it is a pivot around the umbilicus (Wang, J. & Robertson. J, 2008).

Having all these deeply influential points, highlights the energetic importance of the abdomen in relation to the Triple Burner and its vital roles in the body. Along with these influential points there are the AA special Ab points (See chapter 4, *Points on the Abdomen*) which also influence the activities of each of the three Burners through the Bagua blueprint at the earth level of AA.

Through these close links with the Triple Burner, AA has a huge repertoire from which it can exert potentially wide and varied therapeutic effects throughout the whole of the human body.

Meridians of the Abdomen

The abdomen has access to all of the 12 regular channels and collaterals and is also traversed by many of the extraordinary meridians.

The extraordinary meridians are more primal than the ordinary meridians and they exist from the moment the first cell divides. When the ordinary meridians get blocked, it is the extraordinary meridians that ensure that movement continues!

The Ren, Chong and Du Mai originate from the Uterus and give rise to all the other extraordinary meridians that can be manipulated either directly or indirectly via points on the abdomen. Since the point Ren 8 (Shenque) is said to be the mother of all the channels and collaterals, the abdomen has incredible reserves of Qi and Blood. In effect all the meridians can be stimulated through the abdomen either directly or indirectly through the Biao Li (internal: external) connection. So, for example, the Du Mai can be accessed through the Ren Mai and likewise the Kidney meridian can be used to address the Urinary Bladder (UB) meridian.

The Extra Ordinary and Regular Meridians of the Abdomen

- The Ren Mai (Conception Vessel) is also known as the 'Sea of Yin';
- The Du Mai (Governor Vessel) is also known as the 'Sea of Yang';
- The Chong Mai (Penetrating Vessel) is also known as the 'Sea of Blood';
- The Dai Mai (Girdle Vessel) connects all the Vessels;

- The Yin Qiao (Yin Motility Vessel) traverses along the Kid channel (Chace, C. & Shima. M, 2010, p.20);
- The Yin Wei (Yin linking Vessel);
- The Kidney Channel Bi Dimensional connection with UB meridian;
- The Stomach Channel;
- The Spleen Meridian;
- The Liver;
- The Gallbladder.

From this list it is apparent that both Yin and Yang aspects of the meridian system are present on and are accessible through the abdomen. Note the pairings of the extra channels by Li-Shi Zhen, i.e. Ren and Du, Dai and Chong (the Chong Mai is the most internal while the Dai Mai is the most external of the extra meridians).

The Abdomens Special Relationship with the Extra Fu Organs

The six extra Fu organs of the Brain, Gallbladder, Marrow, Bones, Vessels and Uterus can be influenced by various connections with the abdomen, and all have a direct or indirect connection with the Kidneys (Maciocia. G, 2005, pp. 123-125).

The Uterus

The Uterus is located in the lower abdomen, and uterine function is closely related to the Kidney, Ren and Chong meridians. The Ren Mai (Conception Vessel) and the Chong Mai (Penetrating Vessel) originate from the Uterus and so have a huge influence on menstruation, conception/fertility and pregnancy. 'If Kidney Essence is weak the Ren and Chong Mai will be empty and the Uterus will not be supplied with adequate Qi and Blood leading to amenorrhea, irregular cycles and infertility' (Maciocia. G, 2005, pp. 123). The Chong Mai meridian connects with the Kidney meridian from Kid 11 (Hengu) to Kid 21 (Youmen). Kidney 13 (Qixue) and other points along the Kidney meridian at this level can be used to influence both the Chong Mai and the Kidney to improve uterine function.

The Stomach point St 30 (Qichong) connects with another branch of the Chong Mai. This can explain why some women experience nausea and vomiting during menstruation and in pregnancy as a result of changes in the Uterus. Other points in this area of the abdomen, such as Zigong (M-CA-18), will improve Blood and Qi flow and directly influence menstruation, conception and fertility.

The Uterus has a very close functional relationship with Blood, and so normal uterine activity is very much dependant on the Spleen producing enough Blood, the Heart circulating Blood and the Liver storing Blood. Problems with any of these Yin organs can be directly addressed through abdominal acupuncture to ensure normal menstrual cycles and fertility. As Ren 12 (Zhongwan) is at the centre, the middle of the Conception Vessel, it conceivably treats all Yin meridians (Lore, R., 2005).

The term 'Uterus' also applies to men and can be translated as Red Field (Dantian) or the Room of Essence. Male reproductive function is also dependant on strong Kidney Essence and the Du Mai (Governing Vessel). Empty Kidney and Du Mai will result in problems such as impotence, premature ejaculation, watery or clear sperm, nocturnal emissions, spermatorrhoea and other male fertility problems (Maciocia. G, 2005, pp. 124). All these male fertility issues can also be treated well using abdominal acupuncture. Many abdominal prescriptions nourish pre-heaven Qi of the Kidneys with post-heaven Qi from the Spleen (see *chapter 7, Prescriptions: What's the Point?)* thus strengthening the Kidneys to support fertility, conception and pregnancy (abdominal acupuncture is contraindicated during pregnancy).

The Brain

The Brain function is considered to be influenced by many organs including the Kidneys, the Heart and the Liver in particular (see Marrow and Bones below). These meridians are all accessed through the abdomen that makes Brain problems treatable through abdominal acupuncture. In the Spiritual Axis, it is stated in chapter 33 that, 'The Brain is the sea of Marrow extending from the top of the head to the point Feng Fu (Du 16).' The Brain is also influenced by the Du Mai, which has a Biao Li (internal: external) relationship with the Ren Mai, and points such as Du 16 (Fengfu) can be easily stimulated through Ren 11 (Jianli). The image of the turtle has its head in the region of Ren 11(Jianli) and Ren 12 (Zhongwan) allowing this area to treat all Brain problems. The abdomen is known as our second brain with the highest number of neurones outside of the brain and spinal cord. It is also where 95% of serotonin is found and so the abdomen is, therefore, able to address many emotional and psychological conditions such as obsessive–compulsive disorder (OCD), depression and anxiety, (Dr. Keown, D. 2014, p.200) as discussed below.

Marrow and Bone

Both of these are said to be under the jurisdiction of the Kidney. Kidney Essence produces both spinal and Brain Marrow. Marrow develops in Bone cavities and nourishes Bone. Therefore strong Kidney Essence is responsible for both Bone and Marrow production and nourishment. In the *Simple Questions* chapter 34 it states, 'If the Kidneys are deficient, Marrow cannot be abundant'. The Kidneys are particularly well maintained through the function of Ren 6 (Qihai) and Ren 4 (Guanyuan) (see chapter 4, *Points of the Abdomen*).

Abdominal acupuncture prescriptions such as 'Bringing the Qi Home' (see chapter 7, *Prescriptions: What's the Point?*), which has a particular influence on nourishing pre-heaven Qi with post-heaven Qi from the Spleen and the Stomach, ensures that Kidney Essence remains strong to sustain healthy Bones and Marrow.

Blood Vessels

'The Heart dominates the Blood and the Vessels', as stated in the 44th chapter of the ancient writings, Suwen (or 'Plain Questions'). If Heart Qi is strong the Vessels will carry the Blood and remain healthy. The Heart is represented on a number of levels through the abdomen and it can be influenced through the earth (deep) level where the Ba Gua hologram places the Heart at the level of Ren 12 (Zhongwan). The Heart can also be treated through its interaction with the Kidney and the Spleen and often points along the Kidney meridian on the left side are used to treat Heart conditions. The Kidney Essence is also vital as it assists through the production of Marrow, which has a role to play in Blood production. The production of Blood is dependent on the original (Yuan) Qi of the Kidneys (transported by the TB), which contributes to the transformation of food (by the TB) (Gu) Qi into Blood. The abdomen houses a number of influential points (described above) that can directly influence the functions of the TB.

Gallbladder

The Gallbladder meridian passes through the hypochondrium area of the abdomen and is reflected on the Ba Gua as being in the Zhen Gua, which is to the right of the midline. Gallbladder conditions can be treated by needling this area or by using the Liver Qi (elbow) point (Ab1) on the right.

Conventional Modern Scientific Evidence to Support the Power of Abdominal Acupuncture

From a scientific perspective after fertilisation the embryo has three distinctive layers of cells, the ectoderm (relates to the congenital / 1st AMS), the mesoderm and the endoderm. These three layers differentiate into different tissues and organs of the body. The ectoderm forms the skin and the central nervous system (CNS). The mesoderm goes on to form smooth and striated muscle, the circulatory and lymphatic system, Bone and connective tissue. The endoderm forms all the lining of the digestive tract, the bronchioles, Liver and Pancreas and the Urinary Bladder.

The upper and lower limbs start to develop from nodal control centres on the embryo (see Dr. Shang's 'growth control theory of acupuncture' below). During embryonic development there is constant communication between the CNS, skin and limbs. Abdominal acupuncture exploits this close connection and this is one of the mechanisms by which abdominal acupuncture works. Thus by stimulating a point on the abdomen it can have an effect elsewhere on the body. (Tuvla, S. 2008).

Dr. Shang's growth control theory of acupuncture suggests that during embryogenesis, there are nodal areas where there is a high degree of electrical activity. These areas are distributed throughout the body and they act as communication and control centres from which embryo development is orchestrated. Ren 8 (Shenque), is one of these control centres in the abdomen and there are many more along the Ren Mai, and on the abdominal Kidney, Spleen, Stomach and Gall Bladder meridians (Shang, C. 2009). This fact again highlights the importance of the abdomen and is another possible mechanism of understanding the phenomenal power of abdominal acupuncture.

The Abdomen is our Second Brain

Modern science is also recognising the importance of the abdomen in many areas of health, including digestion, immune function, sleep, mood, depression, and even neurological diseases (Hadhazy, A. 2010). The abdomen is often referred to as our second brain because it contains the greatest number of neurones outside of the brain and the spinal cord. It is responsible for the production of many neurotransmitters and hormones such as serotonin.

The gut is where ninety-five percent of serotonin is found (Dr. Keown, D. 2014, p.198) and has a special communication with the brain. The influence of serotonin (the happy hormone) on emotional wellbeing gives the abdomen extra influence on treating emotional conditions such as depression, anxiety and conditions such as obsessive-compulsive disorder (OCD). People suffering from conditions such as depression, OCD and irritable bowel syndrome (IBS) often have a problem with the metabolism of serotonin in the gut being incorrect and therefore causing the levels of serotonin in the brain to change. Serotonin is thus clearly a bowel hormone that affects the brain, as much as the other way around. The abnormal metabolism of serotonin can be addressed specifically by correcting imbalances with the Spleen as the Spleen is responsible for regulating the amount of serotonin circulating in the body through the function of the Blood platelets. Many of the prescriptions used in abdominal acupuncture work directly on the Spleen, such as 'Heaven and Earth' or 'Regulating Spleen Qi' (see, chapter 7, *Prescriptions -What's the Point?*).

I have had quite a lot of success treating the above-mentioned emotional conditions using abdominal acupuncture, and I would postulate that this is as a result of abdominal acupuncture changing the vital serotonin levels so that a more balanced emotional state is achieved.

The abdominal brain makes up the enteric nervous system, which is now recognised as connected to but capable of acting independently from the autonomic nervous system (ANS). The ANS regulates all involuntary activities by affecting smooth muscle, cardiac muscle and glands. It regulates all of the organs including the Heart, Lungs, Uterus, Kidneys, Liver, Stomach, Spleen, eyes and sex organs. The autonomic nervous system is composed of the sympathetic, parasympathetic and enteric nervous systems. The sympathetic and parasympathetic nervous system can increase or decrease activities of organs and have an antagonistic relationship, thus maintaining a homeostatic balance between various organs in the body.

The enteric nervous system controls digestion autonomously by regulating all the gut activity and communicates with the CNS via the para and sympathetic nervous system. Communication between the CNS and the ANS is in a bi-directional manner as described above through the actions of serotonin and its controlling effect on other hormones including insulin!

The abdominal area thus has far-reaching effects on many aspects of human health. These far-reaching and complex effects help to explain some of the therapeutic mechanisms, the diverse side benefits and the incredible potential power of abdominal acupuncture.

Summary of Topics Covered in this Chapter

- The historical importance of the abdomen and it special significance
- The vicinity of the Zang Fu organs with regard to AA points
- The special influence of AA on the Triple Burner
- The regular and extraordinary meridians and the relationship with the abdomen
- The importance of the extraordinary organs and how they affect the abdomens energetics
- Western scientific support to the potential therapeutic power of the abdomen.

Chapter 3: Abdominal Point Location: Get to the Point

Learning Objectives

This chapter details how to locate abdominal acupuncture points using the visual by eye method and using a ruler, which is a more mathematical and formulaic technique. Each system has its merits and these will be discussed so that you can choose whichever technique works best for you. You will learn about the importance of locating the start point correctly with AA so that all other abdominal points are correct. You will also learn about the new abdominal acupuncture (Ab) points as proposed by Professor Bo, which are unique and specific to this system of acupuncture. I will also highlight the patterns that you should look for when using and locating points. This will enable you to recognise at a glance when there is an error in your locations so that it can quickly be corrected. It will also equip you with a more precise and rapid means of finding abdominal Ahshi points.

General Considerations

Abdominal acupuncture point location is important and needs to be very accurate. It is different to conventional acupuncture point location due to the fact that these points represent anatomical areas as represented by the hologram of the turtle. These anatomical areas can be quite small and, therefore, a slight deviation at the beginning can lead to larger errors as you proceed. The unique eight abdominal acupuncture (Ab) points proposed by Professor Bo complete the hologram of the turtle. They include points that represent the elbow (Ab 1), wrist (Ab 2) and thumb (Ab 3) for the upper limb. They also include Ab points below the umbilicus that represent the knee (Ab 4), medial knee (Ab 5), ankle (Ab 6) and sacrum (Ab 7).

Abdominal acupuncture point location uses three distinct and separate methods to locate in different areas of the abdomen, namely:

1. Vertical Superior measurements;
2. Vertical Inferior measurements;
3. Horizontal points measurements.

Because AA is mirroring the anatomy of the body through a hologram of the turtle (at the Heaven / superficial level) the Ren, Stomach and Kidney point locations need to be accurate. The Ren points reflect the location of the head and spine while the location of the Stomach, and particularly the distance to the Kidney meridian, will dictate the measurements for the Ab points, many of which represent the upper and lower limbs.

The three different location zones will often have very different distances for 1 cun, which is unique to that area, i.e. 1 cun in the upper vertical area might be 22 mm while the inferior 1 cun measurement is 32 mm. This is important and will be explained in detail later (see worked example of the formulaic ruler method, section below).

Above the umbilicus, Ren points will often be slightly different to traditional acupuncture point location. This discrepancy is dependent on the distance difference between the xiphisternal synchondrosis and the soft depression of the start point (which are often not the same).

Comparing the Two Systems of Measuring and Locating Abdominal Points

I recommend that you choose whichever method appeals to your particular talents. The ruler method might appeal to someone who is more mathematical while the measurement by eye method might work better for a more visual person! Your confidence locating abdominal points will improve with practice during each new treatment.

I am detailing both location methods to keep this book comprehensive and thus enable you to find the best system for you.

The Merits of Each Method

The choice is yours though the end results should be the same - amelioration of your client's pain. Table 3.1 compares each measuring system.

Measurement by eye	Formulaic Ruler Measurement
Faster	More time consuming especially on 1st visit
Can be less exact when inexperienced	More specific exact locations
No need to carry measurement notes or ruler	Need measurement notes and ruler
Less mathematical	Mathematical formulas can overwhelm

Relies more on patterns	Patterns just confirm correct locations
Better suited to visual people	More suited to mathematically minded
Less worrying /intrusive for client	Ruler can be worrying or intrusive for client

Table 3.1. Comparison of abdominal measurement methods

I personally prefer to locate abdominal points by eye. This is how I was taught in China and in the busy hospital setting where speed was of the essence location by eye was the most efficient method. It is only in recent years with the evolution of AA that measurement with a ruler has been introduced. I have compared measurements using the ruler technique and measurements using my eye and usually there is little or no difference. For this reason I have not seen it necessary to change my method.

If you follow the directions below you will definitely get good results, and you will become more self-assured as a result (more on this subject in chapter 9). So spend the time and get it right from the start.

Protocol for Measuring and Locating Abdominal Points

- It is imperative that your client lies flat with their hands either side of their body. If your client has their hands above their head this will change the location of points;

- When locating points either by eye or using the formulaic ruler method you should stand on the left or right-hand side of the patient parallel with their navel;

- Always strive to keep your head directly above the client's umbilicus. In this way you will see the points and their patterns more correctly (see Fig 3.1);

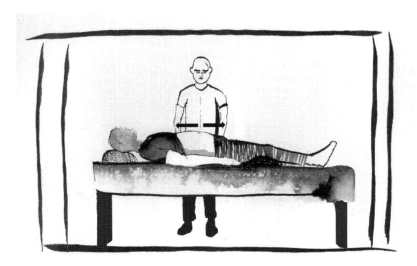

Figure 3.1 Recommended position for client and practitioner

- Avoid stretching or moving the skin as you locate points as this will move the point that you are trying to find. For larger clients with excess skin it may be necessary to move the skin to get a better indication of what the accurate distances from the umbilicus are;

- With larger patients, it may be necessary to place a book or ruler at the flank to get an accurate horizontal measurement. Sometimes rolls of flesh can fall more on one side than the other (see Fig 3.2).

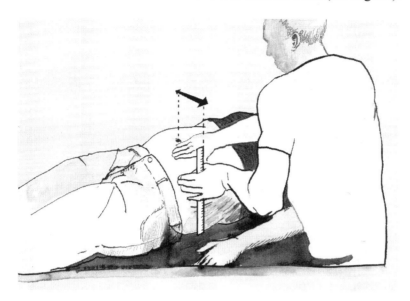

Fig 3.2. How to measure the outer flank accurately with larger clients

- All points should be clearly marked out using iodine or bectotide, which both mark and sterilise at the same time. A non-toxic pen or pencil such as an eyeliner can also be used. Distinctly marking the relevant points will facilitate you seeing the patterns that the different acupuncture points make so that by observation it will become apparent if the point is in the wrong location. Remember that the upper limbs are represented by the hologram of the turtle and should look like an inverted **V**, while the lower limbs should look like a backslash \ (see Fig 3.3).

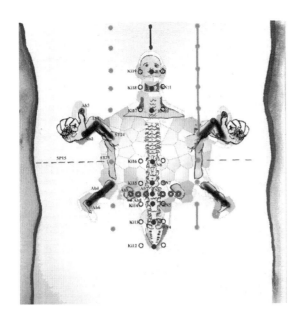

Fig 3.3. The turtle hologram with limb patterns highlighted

Simple Points to Guide you when Locating AA Points Using Either System

Locate the soft depression above the sternum at the xiphisternal synchondrosis. This is the **start point** and must be accurate as all other superior points will be dependent on this measurement.

The start point can be found by sliding your thumbs medially along the exterior borders of the ribs as they arch around the abdomen until they meet in the middle at the bottom of the xiphoid process. Following this, place your thumb on this point and slide it just over the sternum (moving towards the chest) until the pad of your thumb falls into a soft depression that upon palpation will feel tender to your client. This is the start point from which to measure the superior Ren points.

All other Ren points are measured in a similar way to traditional methods and the body units are the same, i.e. it is 8 cun from the centre of the umbilicus to the start point above the sternum, 5 cun to the pubic bone and 6 cun to the outer border on the horizontal measurement.

Special Ab points used to locate all the limb points (Ab 1 to Ab 6) rely on the unique universal ½ cun measurement that is calculated as the distance from the centre of the umbilicus to the Kidney meridian (see below for details). Remember the format of the turtle's fins, as they represent the limbs. The upper limbs (fins) are in the shape of an inverted V, while the lower limbs are in the shape of a \ backslash. (see fig 3.3)

The universal ½ cun measurement is written in this format to distinguish it from a regular half cun measurement, which can change for superior and inferior locations. Use landmark points such as Ren 9 (Shuifen) and Ren 7 (Yinjiao) to help locate shoulder and hip points respectively. Be fluid and trust your client's feedback and/or your intuition to locate Ahshi points.

Tip: When palpating for the border of the pubic bone and the start point be sure to inform clients what you are doing and why. Once they are happy, press through clothing for the pubic bone and if your client is female and you need to put your finger under the front of the bra your client has been informed. Respect your client's dignity at all times.

Option 1: Location Using the Visual Eye Method

Superior Vertical Measurements by Eye

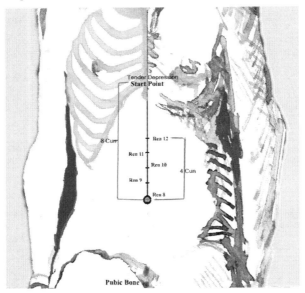

Fig 3.4. Illustration of distance to start point and Ren 12 (Zhongwan)

The distance from the start point above the sternum to the centre of the umbilicus is 8 cun Ren 12 (Zhongwan). It is the uppermost point in abdominal acupuncture and is located 4 cun above Ren 8 (Shenque) (see Fig 3.4).

Ren 12 (Zhongwan) is located by finding the ½ way distance between the tender depression at the start point and the centre of the umbilicus. Use the tip of your index finger and thumb to measure the distance and ensure that this distance is equally divided into 4 cun components (see Fig 3.5).

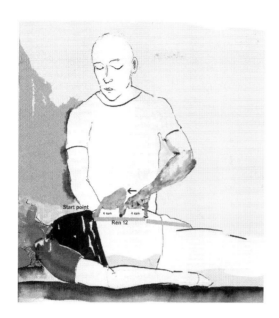

Fig 3.5. Illustration of method for locating Ren 12 by eye

Ren 10 (Xiawan) is the halfway point between, Ren 12 (Zhongwan) and Ren 8 (Shenque), i.e. 2 cun from the centre of the belly button. Again simply use your finger and thumb to get equal distances between these points.

Ren 11(Jianli) is the half way point between Ren 12 (Zhongwan) and Ren 10 (Xiawan). Use your finger and thumb to get equal distances between these points. It is 3 cun superior to the centre of the umbilicus.

Ren 9 (Shuifen) is an important landmark and is the halfway point between the middle of the belly button and Ren 10 (Xiawan). Simply use your finger and thumb to get the 1 cun equal distances between these points.

> **Tip:** Always be methodical about how you locate the points and mark them clearly as described above. In this way you will avoid confusion and potential mistakes.

Horizontal Measurements by Eye

The distance from the centre of the umbilicus to the flank is 6 cun, (see Fig 3.6).

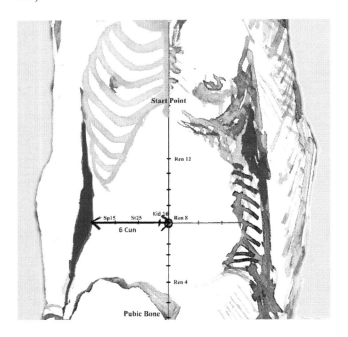

Fig 3.6 Illustration of the AA Horizontal meridian measurements

St 25 (Tianshu) is located by dividing the area from the belly button to the outer limit of the side in three using your index finger and thumb as described above. St 25 (Tianshu) is at the border of the first one-third, i.e. 2 cun lateral to Ren 8 (Shenque).

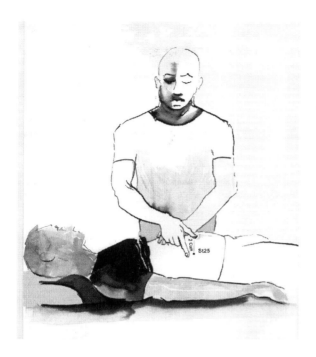

Fig 3.7. Illustration of the visual eye method of locating St 25 (Tianshu)

The Kidney meridian is 0.5 cun lateral to the Ren meridian and is located by dividing the distance to the Stomach points which is 2 cun by 4. To do this by eye, note the halfway mark between the Stomach and Ren meridians and then mark the halfway point between these. This will become second nature in time.

Tip: A cotton bud or Q-tip (used to mark points with iodine) can act as a small ruler to find the half way and then the one-quarter (½ cun) point for the Kidney meridian.

It is important to get this ½ cun measurement as this will act as your **universal ½ cun measurement** necessary for finding Ab points such as elbow, wrist, knee, ankle and the Kidney meridian.

Spleen 15 (Daheng) is found 2 cun lateral to St 25 (Tianshu). It is two-thirds lateral or 4 cun from Ren 8 (Shenque) to the outer flank. Sp 15 (Daheng) is at the border of the abdomonis longis muscle, as in traditional acupuncture point location. Divide the area into thirds using the finger and thumb in a similar way as used to locate St 25 (Tianshu), described above.

When measuring heavier people you may need to use the side of a book or ruler to press against the flank. This can then be used to indicate the outer border of the belly (see Fig 3.2. above).

If the person is quite large sometimes the 6 cun measurement on one side will be greater than that on the other because the body organs are lying more to one side. This discrepancy can alter the location of the horizontal points such as the Stomach, Spleen and to a lesser extent the Kidney meridian points.

When this is the case, it is important that you average out the distance to the Stomach 25 (Tianshu) and Spleen 15 (Daheng) points. In other words, it should be the same distance on either side for the purpose of locating points on the Stomach meridian (see Fig. 3.17) in exact measurement. I have clients in my clinic in whom the difference can be over 30 mm in the 6 cun measurement between one side and the other. This could lead to a difference of 10 mm when measuring St 25 on one side compared to the other!

Inferior Vertical Measurements by Eye

The distance between the centre of the umbilicus and the border of the pubic bone is 5 cun. Measurements below the umbilicus are located by first dividing this distance into five. This can be done using whatever method you usually use to locate the Conception Vessel (Ren) points when locating them for traditional acupuncture.

The distance from the top of the pubic bone to the centre of the umbilicus is 5 cun. Ren 4 (Guanyuan) is 3 cun or three-fifths the way down from the umbilicus. This can be measured by using the piano fingers method. My location method is to divide this 5 cun area in half (i.e. 2.5 cun) using the index finger and thumb in a similar manner to that shown above in Fig. 3.5 and to estimate the other 0.5 cun to give you the 3 cun measurement required for Ren 4 (Guanyuan);

Ren 6 (Qihai) is the midpoint between Ren 4 (Guanyuan) and the umbilicus. This area can be divided into equal (1.5 cun) sections using the index finger and thumb method described above. Alternatively it is halfway between where the second and third fingers lie when dividing the 5 cun into equal parts using piano fingers!

Ren 7 (Yinjiao) is 1 cun below the centre of the umbilicus that is equivalent to two-thirds of the distance to Ren 6 (Qihai). Therefore, simply divide this area into thirds using the finger and thumb or visually locate where the outer border of the second third is. Another method is to simply use the Q-tip as a ruler (as described above to locate the Kidney meridian for the universal ½ cun measurement) to divide the area into thirds. Alternatively Ren 7 (Yinjiao) can be located using the piano fingers method, i.e. where the second finger rests.

It is useful to locate Ren 7 (Yinjiao) which is at the same level and acts as a landmark for locating Stomach 26 (Wailing) or the hip point.

Abdominal point (Ab 7) Qipang is along the Kidney meridian ½ cun (the universal ½ cun) lateral to point Ren 6 (Qihai). This point is anatomically equivalent to the start of the sacrum. All other (abdominal) Kidney points above and below the navel are also found **using the universal ½ cun measurement.**

Locating the Lower Limbs by Eye

When locating points of the leg, hip (St 26 Wailing), knee (Ab 4) and ankle (Ab 6) these should form the shape of a backslash \. See Fig. 3.8.

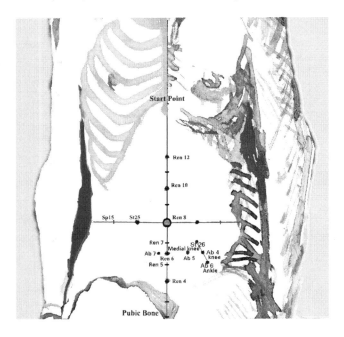

Fig 3.8. Illustration of lower limb point patterns and related Ab points

The hip is located at Stomach 26 (Wailing), which is on a vertical line 1 cun inferior to St 25 (Tianshu) and is at the intersection of the horizontal line with point Ren 7 (Yinjiao).

The knee point (Ab 4) is a half cun inferior (half cun on the Ren line) and a ½ cun lateral to the hip point (N.B. use the universal ½ cun measurements obtained from the horizontal measurements, i.e. it is one-quarter of the distance from the centre of the navel to St 25 Tianshu). The knee point (Ab 4) will be at the intersection of the horizontal line at the same level to point Ren 6 (Qihai) and the vertical line from the elbow (Ab 1) to the knee.

The ankle (Ab 6) then is a half cun inferior and a ½ cun lateral (the universal ½ cun) from the knee. To complete the image of the backslash \ the ankle point (Ab 6) should be on the same vertical line as the wrist above and it should be on a horizontal line with Ren 5 (Shi Men). (See Fig. 3.9).

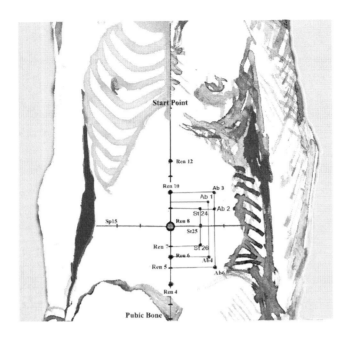

Start Point

Ren 12

Ren 10   Ab 3
          Ab 1
          Ab 2
          St 24
Sp15   Ren 8
          St25
Ren 7   St 26
        Ren 6
        Ab4
Ren 5   Ab6

Ren 4

Pubic Bone

Fig 3.9. The correct alignment of limb points to illustrate patterns formed

The medial knee Ab 5 is located on a line with Ab 4 (knee) back towards the midline up to 1 cun. See turtle hologram, Fig 3.8 and 3.9, (Note this 1 cun area should cater for all over knee problems).

> **Tip:** In clinical practice I have found that most knee problems will be within 0.5 cun medial to the Ab 4 point, i.e. directly 0.5 cun inferior to St 26 (Wailing).

It is important to visualise these imaginary lines so that the tapestry of AA is always apparent and obvious. The foot and toes can be found inferior and medially to the ankle Ab 6 point. Ahshi points for feet will usually be found in this area within a 0.5 cun area (visualise it as if the feet were quite turned in! See Fig. 3.11).

Locating the Upper Limbs by Eye

The shoulder point is St 24 (Huaroumen), which is lateral to Ren 9 (Shuifen) and is superior to and on a vertical line with St 25 (Tianshu).

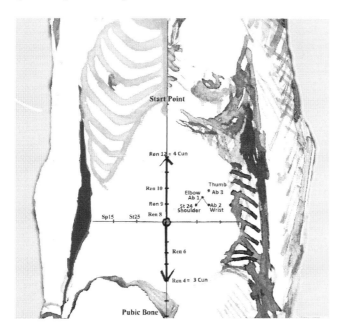

Fig. 3.10. Illustration of upper limb point patterns

The elbow point Ab 1 is a half cun (on the Ren line) superior and ½ cun (universal ½ cun measurement) lateral to St 24 (Huaroumen). It should be on a line half way between Ren 9 (Shuifen) and Ren 10 (Xiawan).

The wrist point Ab 2 is a half cun inferior and a ½ cun (universal) lateral to Ab 1, i.e. it is 1 cun lateral to St 24 (Huaroumen). The shoulder, elbow (Ab 1) and wrist (Ab 2) should resemble an inverted **V** (just like the upper fins of a turtle) (see Fig 3.10 above).

The thumb point Ab 3 is 1 cun directly superior to the wrist point Ab 2. The tip of the thumb should be on a horizontal line level with Ren 10 (Xiawan).

To locate the fingers, these will be found lateral (approximately within a distance of about 0.5 cun) and superior to the wrist, and to a level as high as the elbow Ab 1 point (see Fig. 3.11).

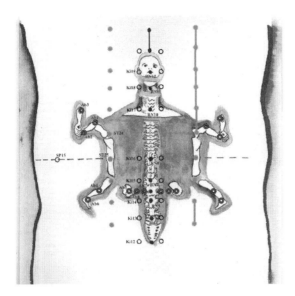

Fig. 3.11. The turtle hologram

Tip: Remain focused as you locate landmarks. Make a mental note of these and for what points they are landmarks. As you add points, such as shoulder St 24 (Huaroumen) or knee (Ab 4), take a moment to observe. Check they are in line with the landmarks and whether they make the patterns they should (see Figs. 3.8, 3.9 and 3.10). If not, why not? Fix and continue.

Option 2: AA Point Location Mathematical Formulaic Method

Exact Formulaic Abdominal Measurements General Considerations

When using this more mathematical formulaic method measure in millimetres (mm). Anything smaller than that should be rounded off. The location of points when there are small discrepancies will be obvious by the presence of Ahshi points. Use a clear plastic ruler with millimetre (mm) markings. Millimetre markings are less likely to get confused with cun figures than (centimetre) cm when keeping records.

I recommend that you highlight important figures such as the universal ½ cun measurement and the lower and upper vertical 1 cun measurements, as these will be referred to when measuring out the upper and lower limbs (see Fig. 3.21 and Appendix for blank record chart fig A5). It will make you less prone to mistakes while ensuring measuring out and marking your patients is much more accurate. Remember these measurements will remain the same for your client's future visits (unless they increase or decrease their weight dramatically) and minutes spent meticulously getting the figures correct and making good records will save you time in the long run.

Some Special Considerations when Locating Points using Formulaic Ruler Method

Using a ruler with a client can be awkward so use these simple suggestions to avoid un- necessary upset to your client:

It is important to position the ruler so that the 0 mm marking is at the start point (above the sternum) or from the top Ren point located and directed inferiorly towards the centre of the umbilicus when measuring the upper vertical zones. This will prevent the ruler going up towards the face and irritating your client. Position the 0 mm ruler marking at the centre of the umbilicus when doing horizontal measurements. That way you can use the edge of the book or ruler pressed against the clients flank to give an accurate measurement (see Fig. 3.12).

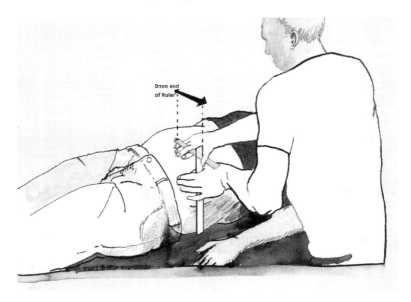

0mm end
of Ruler

Fig 3.12. The ruler start point for measuring the horizontal points

Avoid the ruler going too far down your clients groin area. It's better to use the upper border of the pubic area as the 0 mm ruler start point when measuring the inferior vertical points.

Worked Examples of the Formulaic Ruler Method

Exact Formulaic Abdominal Measurements for the Upper Vertical Zone

Use the same process as described above in 'simple points to guide you when locating AA points', using either system to locate the 'tender to the touch' start point just above the sternum at the xiphisternal synchondrosis.

If the distance from the start point (i.e. the sensitive depression just above the sternum) to the middle of the navel is 180 mm **(i.e. 8 cun = 180 mm)** then divide this by 2 to give the exact distance to Ren 12 (Zhongwan) **(i.e. 4 cun) 180 mm ÷ 2 = 90 mm** (see Fig. 3.13). Or simply calculate the 1 cun figure by dividing the 8 cun figure by 8, **i.e. 180 mm ÷ 8 = 22.5 mm, i.e. 1 cun, 22.5 x 4 = 90mms,** i.e. Ren 12 (Zhongwan). This 1 cun figure can be used to calculate all other upper Ren points as described below.

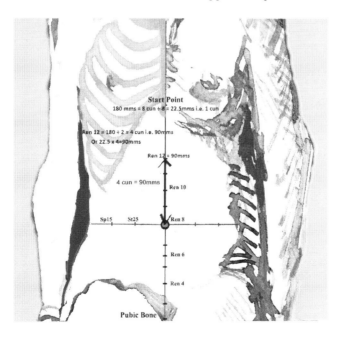

Fig. 3.13. How to measure exact location of Ren 12 (Zhongwan)

The measurement for Ren 11 (Jianli) is found by simply multiplying the 1 cun figure of 22.5 mm by 3, i.e. **22.5 mm x 3 = 67.5 mm** (round down to 67 mm) (see Fig. 3.14).

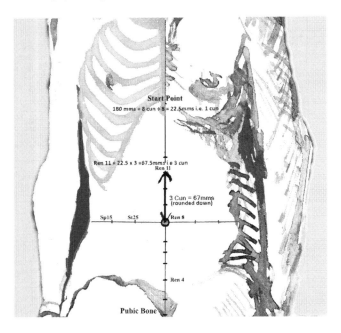

Fig. 3.14. How to measure exact location of Ren 11 (Jianli)

To calculate the distance to Ren 10 (Xiawan) multiply the 1 cun figure by 2, i.e. **22.5 mm x 2 = 45 mm**. Alternatively, divide the Ren 12 (Zhongwan) figure by 2 to give the same result i.e. **90 mm ÷ 2 = 45 mm or 2 cun** (see Fig. 3.15).

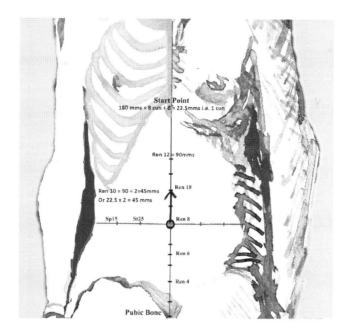

Fig. 3.15. How to measure exact location of Ren 10 (Xiawan)

Finally, either divide this 2 cun figure by 2 to get the distance to Ren 9 (Shuifen) and for St 24 (Huaroumen) points, i.e. **45 mm ÷ 2 = 22.5 mm**, or simply use the 1 cun figure you have from earlier (round this figure off to 22 mm or 23 mm) equals **1 cun** (see Fig. 3.16).

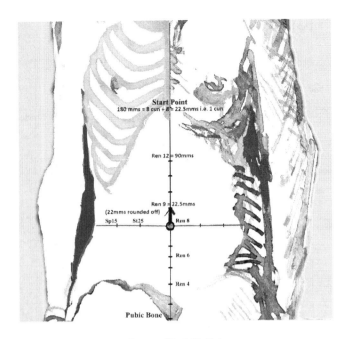

Fig. 3.16 How to measure exact location of Ren 9 (Shuifen)

Exact Formulaic Abdominal Measurements for the Horizontal Zone

Be aware that the sides of some people may have different measurements so use an average for each side. For example, The left side measures 180 mm, i.e. 6 cun and the right side measurement is 200 mm, which is also 6 cun, therefore the figure used for each side is **180 + 200 = 380 ÷ 2 = 190 mm** (see Fig. 3.17).

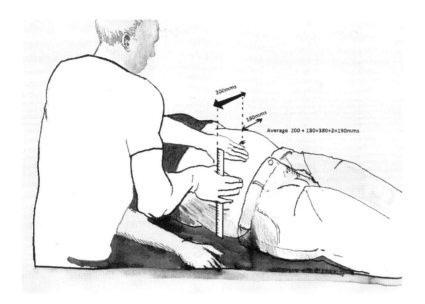

Fig. 3.17. How to measure average horizontal distance in larger clients

When measuring large, heavier people you may need to use the side of a book or a ruler to press against the flank. This can then be used to indicate the outer border and will be easily measured on the ruler (see Fig. 3.18).

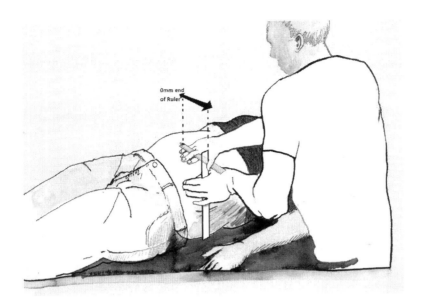

Fig. 3.18. How to accurately measure larger clients' horizontal region

The area from the centre of the umbilicus to the flank is **6 cun,** which in this example is 150 mm. Therefore to get the distance to St 25 (Tianshu) divide this figure by 3, e.g. **150 mm ÷ 3 = 50 mm i.e. 2 cun** (see Fig. 3.19).

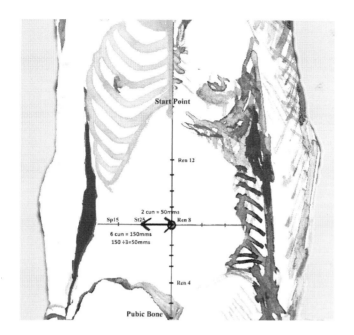

Fig 3.19. How to measure exact location of St 25 (Tianshu)

To get the **universal ½ cun** measurement, divide the 2 cun figure by 4, i.e. **50 mm ÷ 4 = 12.5 mm.** This figure can be rounded off, either up or down (see Fig 3.20).

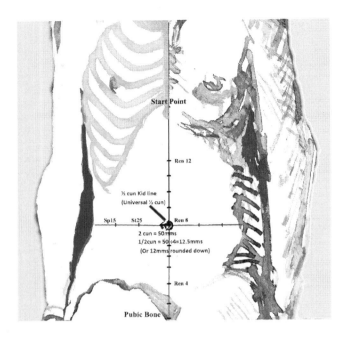

Fig. 3.20. Exact measurement for the Kidney meridian and the universal ½ cun

The horizontal ½ cun acts as the universal measurement above and below the central Ren 8 (Shenque), keep this universal ½ cun figure highlighted for simplicity (see Fig. 3.21).

Tip: Use a record sheet such as Fig. 3.21 below and highlight the important figures such as the universal ½ cun measurement, the superior and inferior 1 cun measurement. Clarity will stand to you especially in the early days when you have a list of different figures relating to different cun measurements in different abdominal zones.

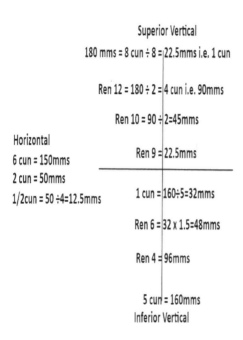

Superior Vertical

180 mms = 8 cun ÷ 8 = 22.5mms i.e. 1 cun

Ren 12 = 180 ÷ 2 = 4 cun i.e. 90mms

Ren 10 = 90 ÷ 2=45mms

Horizontal

6 cun = 150mms

2 cun = 50mms

1/2cun = 50 ÷4=12.5mms

Ren 9 = 22.5mms

1 cun = 160÷5=32mms

Ren 6 = 32 x 1.5=48mms

Ren 4 = 96mms

5 cun = 160mms

Inferior Vertical

Fig. 3.21. Example of a record sheet for formulaic measurements

Spleen 15 (Daheng) is located as being two-thirds the way or 4 cun from the centre of the umbilicus to the outer border of the flank. Or it is at the border of the abdomonis longis muscle, where this is visible. Therefore **150 mm is divided by 3 and multiplied by 2 to give 100 mm.** Or simply multiply the 2 cun figure used to locate St 25 (Tianshu) by 2 to give 4 cun, i.e. **50 mm x 2 = 100 mm** the distance to Sp 15 (Daheng) (see Fig. 3.22).

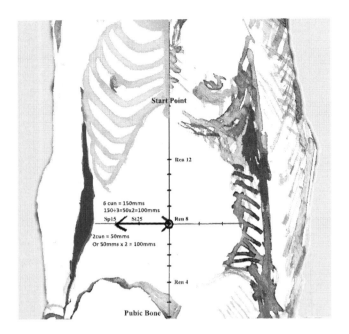

Fig 3.22 How to get the exact measurement for Sp 15 (Daheng)

Exact Formulaic Abdominal Measurements for the Inferior Vertical Zone

The distance from the navel to the pubic bone is 5 cun which is 160 mm for this example. To get the 1 cun figure divide the distance 160 mm by 5, **160 mms ÷ 5 = 32 mm (1 cun).**

> **Tip:** This 1 cun measurement should also be highlighted for finding Ren 7 (Yinjiao), which will act as a landmark for Stomach 26 (Wailing), i.e. hip points.

Ren 4 (Guanyuan) is calculated by multiplying this 1 cun figure by 3, **i.e. 32 mm x 3 = 96 mm**. Therefore **Ren 4 (Guanyuan) is 96 mm** below the centre of the umbilicus (see Fig. 3.23).

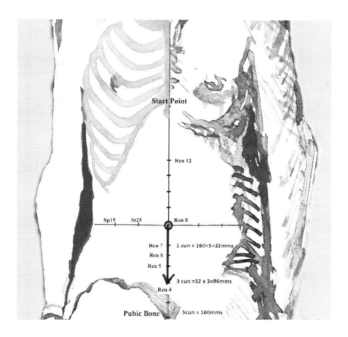

Fig. 3.23 How to get the exact measurement for Ren 4 (Guanyuan)

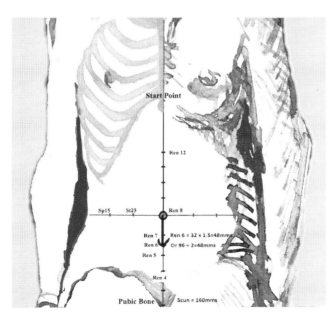

Ren 6 (Qihai) is half of **96 mms ÷ 2 = 48 mms.** Alternatively just multiply the 1 cun figure by 1.5, i.e. **32 x 1.5 = 48 mms** (see Fig. 3.24).

Fig. 3.24. How to get the exact measurement for Ren 6 (Qihai)

Locating the Lower Limb points using the Ruler Method

The hip point St 26 (Wailing) is **1 cun, i.e. 32 mm** below St 25 (Tianshu) (see Fig. 3.25).

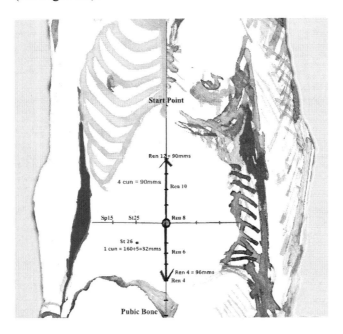

Fig. 3.25. How to get the exact location of St 26 (Wailing)

The ½ cun for the knee (Ab 4) and ankle (Ab 6) **lateral** measurements uses the **universal ½ cun measurement of 12.5mms** *(N.B. this is the unique universal ½ cun measurement of 12.5mms obtained from the Kidney meridian measurements),* which can be rounded up or down. (See Fig. 3.26).

The half cun used for the knee (Ab 4) and ankle (Ab 6) **inferior** measurements use the half cun measurements along the inferior Ren meridian. In other words the hip is level with Ren 7 (Yin Jiao), the knee is level with Ren 6 (Qihai), and the ankle is level with Ren 5 (Shi Men), as illustrated in Fig. 3.26.

The knee Ab 4 is located 12 mm (the universal ½ cun, measurement) lateral and a half cun (on the Ren meridian) inferior to St 26 (Wailing) on a line level with Ren 6 (Qihai) and on a vertical line level with the elbow (Ab 1) point.

The ankle point Ab 6 is on a line 12 mm (universal ½ cun) lateral and a half cun (on the Ren meridian) inferior to the knee point Ab 4. The ankle Ab 6 point is on a vertical line level with the wrist Ab 2. Hip, knee and ankle points should look like a backslash \ (see Fig. 3.26 and fig 3.28).

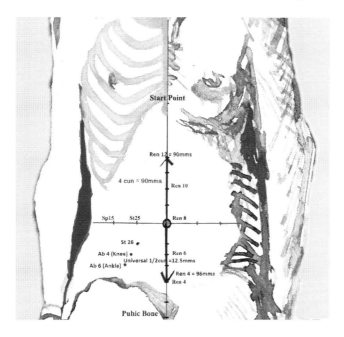

Fig. 3.26. How to locate Ab 4 (knee) and Ab 6 (ankle) points

The medial knee point (Ab 5) is 24 mm or 1 cun (i.e. the universal 1/2 cun, rounded down figure of 12 mm multiplied by 2) medial to the knee point Ab 4.

Tip: In clinical practice I have found that most knee problems will be within 0.5 cun (12 mm) medial to the Ab 4 point, i.e. directly 0.5 cun inferior to St 26 (Wailing).

Points for the foot and toes are located medially and inferior to the ankle Ab 6 and should be within a 0.5 cun radius of this area.

Locating the Upper Limb Points using the Ruler Method

When locating points shoulder St. 24 (Huaroumen) elbow (Ab 1) and wrist (Ab 2) points these should form the shape of an inverted **V**. The shoulder is located at Stomach 24 (Huaroumen) which is on a vertical line 1 cun superior to Stomach 25 (Tianshu) and is at the intersection of a horizontal line with point Ren 9 (Shuifen).

The elbow point (Ab 1) is a half cun (on the Ren meridian) superior and 12mms (the universal ½ cun) lateral to the shoulder point. The elbow point (Ab 1) will be at the intersection of an imaginary horizontal line at the halfway level between Ren 9 (Shuifen) and Ren 10 (Xiawan).

The wrist (Ab 2) point is half a cun (on the Ren meridian as distinct from the universal ½ cun measurement) inferior and 12 mm (universal ½ cun) lateral to the elbow (Ab 1), completing the image of the inverted **V** that is the shape of the turtle's front fin. The wrist point should be on the same vertical line as the ankle below, and it should be on a horizontal line level with the shoulder and Ren 9 (Shuifen) (see Fig. 3.27 & 3.28).

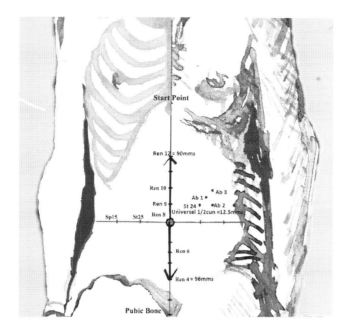

Fig. 3.27. How to get the exact location of upper limb points

The thumb point Ab 3 is 1 cun superior to the wrist Ab 2 point and should be on a line level with Ren 10 (Xiawan) see fig 3.27 and 3.28.

Finger points are located within an area of approximately 0.5 cun lateral and superior to the wrist Ab 2 point. Use Ahshi points to direct you.

> **Tip:** Don't be intimidated by the maths. Take a breather, be systematic, and it will all make sense!

The same abdominal patterns should be obvious with this more mathematical way of locating points (see Fig. 3.28). It is good practice to see these patterns every time you use abdominal acupuncture so that errors will be recognised and Ahshi points isolated rapidly.

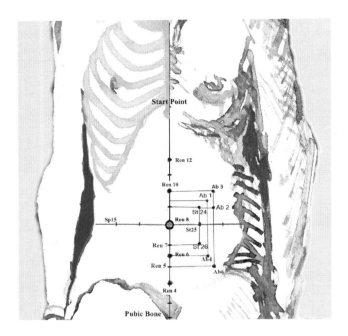

Labels in figure: Start Point, Ren 12, Ren 10, Ab 3, Ab 1, St 24, Ab 2, Sp15, Ren 8, St25, Ren 7, St 26, Ren 6, Ab4, Ren 5, Ab6, Ren 4, Pubic Bone

Fig. 3.28. The correct alignment of limb points & patterns formed.

Build on the Bones of the Turtle

There is a famous saying in Chinese medicine 'Jian Yi' which translates as simplicity. This is a useful thing to remember when treating someone with abdominal acupuncture. No matter what your treatment always mark out the Bones of the turtle. Once you have these, then you can add the flesh for more focused treatments.

1. Accurately isolate the sensitive to touch **start point** for the superior vertical measurements;

2. Locate and mark all the main **Superior Ren** points including 12 (Zhongwan), 10 (Xiawan) and 9 (Shuifen). Note the anatomical significance of each point and the important relevant landmarks;

3. Next locate and mark all the main **Inferior Ren** points including Ren 7 (Yinjiao), Ren 6 (Qihai) and Ren 4 (Guanyuan). Once again make a reference of the anatomical significance of each point and the important landmarks;

4. Locate and mark St 25 (Tianshu) and any other relevant Stomach points for hip, shoulder or, if using the abdominal, four gates. Having St 24 (Huaroumen) and St 26 (Wailing) marked out also makes locating elbow (Ab 1), wrist (Ab 2), knee (Ab 4) and ankle (Ab 6) easier to do (see Fig. 3.28).

Once you have the skeleton of the turtle the patterns of this beautiful tapestry will become obvious and it will be easier to locate Ahshi points for the conditions being treated. For instance, if treating a right lateral elbow problem, once you have right Ab 1 (elbow) marked it is easier to locate and mark Ahshi points (nodes) in the area and focus the treatment in order to fix the problem.

Tip: Avoid the temptation to do what students on my courses often do initially, which is to get too excited when presented with a case and mark up lots of unnecessary points. This will result in all important patterns getting lost in a dot-to-dot series like a child's drawing game! By all means get excited by the challenge presented by each case but maintain your concentration and be methodical.

The Tapestry of the Turtle will be your Guide

Once you are confident locating AA points, the patterns will jump out at you and they will be your guide. Soon you will find that you can pinpoint

Ahshi points in a matter of minutes. If you find that the formulaic ruler system works for you, then use it. Once you have got the figures for a client, they will not change unless they dramatically increase or decrease their weight. If you keep those measurements, then you should be able to mark the point locations on subsequent visits almost as fast as doing it by eye.

The advantage of doing it by eye is that you don't need to have your notes or a ruler to do a treatment. The most important thing is that you get good results from the very first time you use abdominal acupuncture. If the results are not what you expect then look at the patterns, check measurements and review the depths of needles. (See chapter 9, *Putting it all Together*).

Summary of Topics Covered in this Chapter

- The importance of locating the correct start point
- The three different measuring zones, namely superior and inferior vertical and horizontal
- A comparison of the two point location methods
- The protocol for client and practitioner for accurate point location
- A step-by-step system for measuring all AA points by eye
- Detailed worked examples of locating AA points using the formulaic mathematical ruler method
- A brief synopsis of how to construct the turtle.

Chapter 4: Points on the Abdomen

Learning Objectives

In this chapter we will revise the main Jing Lou/traditional acupuncture points used and the new abdominal acupuncture (Ab) points that are specific to this system. We will discuss each point's functions in respect to traditional and abdominal acupuncture. Each point will also be described in relation to its anatomical position when it is represented by the turtle/tortoise hologram. General location is given here but for a more detailed explanation of how to locate abdominal points see the previous chapter, *Abdominal Point Location: Get to the Point*. Needle depths will be suggested for treating different conditions.

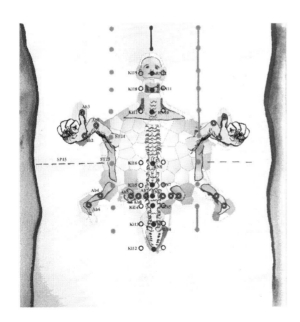

Fig 4.1. Hologram of the AA turtle

General Considerations

As acupuncturists I am aware that you will be familiar with the functions of many of the abdominal points mentioned. I feel that it is beneficial to appreciate the function of and the special nature of many of the points involved in abdominal acupuncture. Equally, a review of each point's relevance helps to paint a picture of how these commonly used points can exert such powerful effects. Frequently my clients report some profound responses to AA. It is only apparent after reviewing the nature of the acupuncture point and its interactions with other points or meridians that a mechanism by which such diverse reactions occur can be explained.

My clients often declare that they have much better energy levels, their sleep has improved, blood pressure has, 'decreased to the best consistent levels in years', their mood has improved and that anxiety levels have reduced dramatically following a couple of AA treatments. I realise that these are benefits that are also frequently seen with traditional acupuncture but with AA the degree and variety of changes seem to be far greater.

Please note that point function references have come from a number of sources (Deadman, P. et al 2011; Pedersen, R.M, 2002, pp.36-37, 46, 76-77, 106-111; Giovanni, M. 2005. pp.385-387, 430-432, 460-464), Yang C. 2012 and Dr. Han Yan personal communication 2004).

CASE STUDY: Full of Dampness

A client in her early 70's had Cold Damp Bi Syndrome with joint pain, especially in her knees and elbows. She was suffering from an acute attack of a chronic sinusitis problem too, which was giving her a frontal headache and making it difficult to breathe through her nose. She had a heaviness about her limbs, and she described her energy levels as very low. She also had osteoporosis.

Her daughter, a doctor, had prescribed antibiotics for the sinusitis and wanted her to go on various other medications. However, she was reluctant to do so as it might cloud her daily meditation practice.

I used AA prescription of 'Guiding Qi Home', i.e. Ren 12 (Zhongwan), Ren 10 (Xiawan), Ren 6 (Qihai) and Ren 4 (Guanyuan). I then reinforced Ren 4 (Guanyuan) with bilateral Kid 13 (Qixue) and I needled 'Feng Shi Dian' bilateral, upper rheumatism (Ab 1) elbow points and upper lateral rheumatism (Ab 2), wrist points, lower rheumatism (Ab 4) knee points and lower lateral rheumatism (Ab 6) ankle points. I also used St 24 (Huaroumen) and a special point for treating the sinuses 0.2 cun inferior and medial to St 24 (Huaroumen). I finally included Sp 15 (Daheng) to clear Damp, ease pain and lubricate the joints (see Fig 4.2).

I checked how the pain in the knees was, and it was completely gone, with more mobility there also. The sinuses felt clearer, and I encouraged her to breathe through her nose so that she would benefit from the production of nitric oxide. This acts as a broncho-dilator and has antibacterial and antiviral properties.

On her next visit she was very happy with the progress. Her energy levels had dramatically improved, the heaviness and stiffness in the joints were reduced by 60-70%, and her sinus headache was gone. She declared that the benefits from AA were far superior to any other acupuncture treatments she had received previously.

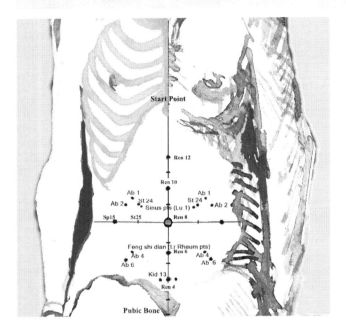

Fig 4.2. AA Prescription for case history 'Full of Dampness'

Abdominal Points

Ren 12 (Zhongwan) 'Middle Epigastrium'

Functions of Ren 12 (Zhongwan)

Front Mu pt. of the St. Hui meeting point of the Fu organs:

- Meeting pt. of the Ren, Small Intestine, Stomach, Lung and San Jiao meridians;
- Harmonises the middle Jiao and descends rebellious Qi;

~ 112 ~

- Tonifies the St and fortifies the Sp;
- Tonifies Qi;
- Resolves Dampness;
- Regulates Qi and alleviates pain;
- Treats all diseases of the Spleen and Stomach, including those arising due to injury by any of the seven emotions, which can lead to epigastric pain;
- It is one of the cardinal points of the Ren Mai which stimulates the upper abdomen and Yang organs.

Ren 12 (Zhongwan) Abdominal Significance

- Head of the turtle/tortoise specifically located as the mouth area;
- Treats head, Brain and sense organs (Ahshi) at the heaven / superficial level (Fig 4.1);
- Affects internal organs Sp/St., Heart and SI (Earth deep level).

Point Location

Ren 12 (Zhongwan)

Located halfway between depression above the top of the sternum and the centre of umbilicus/Ren 8 (Shenque).

When treating sense organs, these might be located within the area to a radius of 0.5-1.0 cun superior and or lateral to Ren 12 (Zhongwan).

Needling Depths for Different Conditions

To treat sense organs or skin problems very superficial needling is used (0.1-0.2 cun).

When treating a frontal headache the depth is more superficial 0.1-0.3 cun than an occipital headache that may be to a depth of approximately 0.4 cun (Fig 4.3). See case histories, 'A Total Headcase' and 'Headaches from Hell', in chapter 8, *Abdominal Acupuncture Prescriptions for Frequently seen Painful Conditions*.

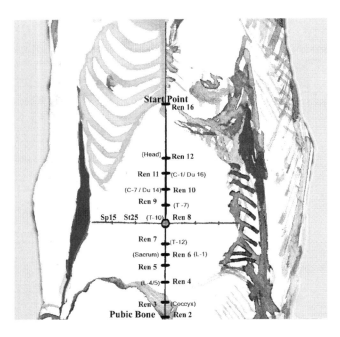

Fig 4.3. Chart of main Ren points and anatomical significance in AA

Ren 11 (Jianli) 'Building Mile'

Functions of Ren 11 (Jianli)

- Harmonises the middle Jiao and regulates Qi;
- Promotes digestion and stimulates the descending of Stomach Qi;
- Especially good for food Stagnation;
- Treats abdominal distension.

Ren 11 (Jianli) Abdominal Significance

- Is anatomically equivalent to point Du 16 (Feng Fu/sea of Marrow) (Fig 4.3);
- Treats problems at cervical vertebra No.1;
- Used for Brain problems and, like Du 16 (Feng Fu), should only be needled superficially;
- It can be used to clear internal or external Wind and can treat conditions such as dizziness, tremor, Wind stroke and Parkinson's disease.

Point Location

Ren 11 (Jianli) is located 1 cun, inferior to Ren 12 (Zhongwan) along the midline. It is 3 cun superior to Ren 8 (Shenque).

Needling Depths for Different Conditions

When treating problems with the throat, if they are more frontal then superficial needling is required 0.1-0.2 or 0.3 cun. Skin problems are needled to a depth of 0.1 cun or less. When working on cervical vertebra problems depth can be up to 0.3 to 0.5 cun. See, case history, 'A Busy Chef's Neck and Shoulder Pain' in chapter 8, *Abdominal Acupuncture Prescriptions for Frequently seen Painful Conditions*.

Caution should be observed when needling this point that it is not needled deeper than approximately 0.5 cun. This is also the case when needling the point Du 16 (Feng Fu) in conventional body acupuncture. It can be dangerous to needle deeper! (Dr. Han Yan. Personal communication 2002)

Ren 10 (Xiawan) 'Lower Epigastrium'

Functions of Ren 10 (Xiawan)

- Ren 10 (Xiawan) is the meeting point of the Ren and Spleen meridians;
- It harmonises the Stomach and regulates Qi;
- Tonifies the Spleen;
- Especially good for moving and tonifying;
- Dispels food Stagnation.

Ren 10 (Xiawan) Abdominal Significance

- This point is level with the spinous process of cervical vertebra no.7 (C-7);
- Just below this point 1 fen (1/10 of a cun) is anatomically equivalent to Du 14 (Dahzui);

- Helps Ren 12 (Zhongwan) acts as a minister point for Sp. and St. conditions;
- Du 14 (Dahzui), 'Sea of Qi', is just below Ren 10 (Xiawan). It can be used to treat a cold due to Wind Heat.

Point Location

Ren 10 (Xiawan) is the half way point between Ren 12 (Zhongwan) and the centre of Ren 8 (Shenque), it is 2 cun above Ren 8 (Shenque).

Needling Depths for Different Conditions

Throat problems can be treated between Ren 11 (Jianli) and Ren 10 (Xiawan) and are usually needled less deeply, i.e. 0.1 - 0.3 cun, if there is an Ahshi point present. This will be represented by a node or resistant point. Needle through it and come back to the original depth where the resistance first appeared. Vertebra problems should be needled to a level of 0.3 - 0.5 cun. When treating Wind Heat at the acute phase, needle 0.1 cun (1 fen) below Ren 10 (Xiawan) to stimulate the point Du 14 (Dahzui). The depth should be at approximately 0.5-0.7 cun. Whereas when treating dizziness and/or tremors deeper needling to a depth of 0.7-1.2 cun will give better results (Fig 4.3).

Ren 9 (Shuifen) 'Water Separation'

Functions of Ren 9 (Shuifen)

- Meeting point of the Ren and Lung meridian;
- Promotes the separation of fluids;
- Regulates the water passages and treats oedema especially (Yin type) when due to Kid and Sp Deficiency;
- Treats the manifestations of Damp;
- Harmonises the intestines and dispels accumulation;
- Acts on the middle Burner together with Ren 12 (Zhongwan).

Ren 9 (Shuifen) Abdominal Significance

- Ren 9 (Shuifen) is anatomically equivalent to thoracic vertebra no. 7 (T-7);
- This point should be needled for acute back and neck ache;
- It helps reduce swelling at the acute stage of back pain;
- Can be particularly effective for treating herniated or slipped disc's.

Point Location

Ren 9 (Shuifen) is located either half way between Ren 10 (Xiawan) and Ren 8 (Shenque) or is 1 cun above Ren 8 (Shenque). See Fig 4.3.

Needling Depths for Different Conditions

This point is often used to reduce swelling in the case of an acute back or neck sprain. In this situation it should be needled to a depth of between

0.6-1.0 cun. When treating thoracic vertebra no.7 the depth is usually approximately 0.5 cun (see Fig. 4.3). For reference, look at case histories 'A Dancer's Potential Disaster', 'Sneezed and Seized' and 'Maddening Mastitis' in chapter 8, *Abdominal Acupuncture Prescriptions for Frequently Seen Painful Conditions*.

Ren 8 (Shenque) 'Spirit Gate'

Functions of Ren 8 (Shenque)

- This point is never needled but can be stimulated with moxa to warm and raise the Yang;
- Yang within Yin expels Cold;
- Rescues Yang;
- Tonifies original Qi.

Ren 8 (Shenque) Abdominal Significance

- This is the source of all the abdominal, regular and extraordinary meridian systems;
- It is at the level of the 10th thoracic vertebrae;
- This is the central point of abdominal acupuncture. It is the mother of the AMS and the Jing Lou meridian systems;
- This is one of the foundations upon which abdominal acupuncture is based.

Point Location

The centre of the umbilicus.

Needling Depths for Different Conditions

No Needling. You can use indirect moxa or moxa cones on ginger to elevate the Yang with sea salt in the umbilicus below the slice of ginger as it clears Damp.

Ren 7 (Yinjiao) 'Yin Crossing'

Functions of Ren 7 (Yinjiao)

- This is the meeting point of the Conception and Penetrating Vessels and the Kidney meridian;
- It regulates menstruation and benefits the lower abdomen and genital region. It is said to treat the lower Burner where the clear and turbid are separated from food and fluid   (Wang, J. & Robertson, J., 2008, p.227);
- Nourishes Yin;
- Influences the Triple Burner.

Ren 7 (Yinjiao) Abdominal Significance

- It is at the level of the 12th thoracic vertebrae;

- It is an important landmark as it is level with St 26 (Wailing), which is the hip point.

Point Location

1 cun inferior to Ren 8

Needling Depths for Different Conditions

Vertebra problems should be needled to a level of 0.3-0.5 cun. When treating frontal problems medial to the hip more superficial needling will be necessary (Fig 4.3).

Ren 6 (Qihai) 'Sea of Qi'

Functions of Ren 6 (Qihai)

- Ren 6 (Qihai) is known as the Sea of Qi;
- It has a powerful tonifying effect on both Qi and Yang;
- Tonifies the original Qi;
- Tonifies the Kidneys and Yang;
- Regulates Qi and harmonises Blood;
- Resolves Dampness;
- Tonifies the Spleen;
- Treats all kinds of chronic Qi disease;
- It is one of the cardinal points of the Ren Mai which stimulates the lower abdomen, sexual organs and energy levels.

Ren 6 (Qihai) Abdominal Significance

Ren 6 (Qihai) is anatomically level with the 1st lumbar vertebra (L-1).

Ren 6 (Qihai) is often reinforced using Ab 7 (see below) points along the Kidney meridian to invigorate the Spleen to help nourish the muscles and tendons.

Point Location

Ren 6 (Qihai) is the midpoint between Ren 4 (Guanyuan) and the umbilicus, i.e. it is 1.5 cun below Ren 8 (Shenque).

Needling Depths for Different Conditions

When treating vertebra problems, needling is to a depth of 0.5-1.0 cun or even deeper on occasion. To invigorate the Spleen and Kidneys the depth can be up to 1-1.5 cun.

Ren 4 (Guanyuan) 'Gate of the Original Qi'

Functions of Ren 4 (Guanyuan)

- Front Mu point of the Small Intestine;
- Meeting point with the Spleen, Liver and Kidney;
- Tonifies the original Qi and benefits the Essence;
- Tonifies the Kidneys and nourishes the Lung;
- Warms and tonifies the Spleen;
- Regulates the Uterus;
- Strengthens Yang;
- Nourishes Blood and Yin;

- Calms the mind;
- Roots the Ethereal soul;
- Especially good for both male and female fertility problems.

Ren 4 (Guanyuan) Abdominal Significance

- Anatomically relates to lumbar vertebra No.4 or 5;
- Is equivalent to Du 3 (Yaoyangguan);
- The tail of the turtle.

Du 3 (Yaoyangguan) is indicated for any lumbar pain affecting the knees and legs. Ren 3 (Zhongji) is level with the coccyx. Shallow needling just below Ren 4 acts on the external genitals.

Point Location

Ren 4 (Guanyuan) is located by dividing the area between the top of the pubic bone and the umbilicus in five. It is three-fifths or 3 cun inferior to the centre of the umbilicus.

Needling Depths for Different Conditions

When treating vertebra problems needling is to a depth of 0.4-1.0 cun or even deeper on occasion. To invigorate the Kidneys the depth can be up to 1-1.2 cun. The Small Intestine is involved in separating the clear and turbid and assists the Spleen in further classification of nutrients. This, coupled with the fact that it also assists the Heart in making the Blood red by sending nutrients directly through the Heart (its paired organ) Ren 4 (Guanyuan), means it can often be used to treat anaemia and other Blood conditions. (Wang, J. & Robertson, J. 2008, pp. 190-193).

CASE STUDY: Needle Phobic with a Headache

Mary, a wary client with a fear of needles, mentioned on her first visit that she had a severe right-sided headache above and behind her eye.

I explained how gentle AA is and said that I would only use two or three points (I avoided using the word needles for obvious reasons). She was still reluctant, so I asked permission to press her abdomen with a pointed forefinger. This was to indicate the sensation she would feel from acupuncture. I placed my finger around Ren 12 (Zhongwan) and with a quick forward motion depressed in and out approximately a half a cun. I explained that, in the main, this should be all that she would feel!

Having won her confidence I wasted no time and proceeded with the treatment. I located Ren 12 (Zhongwan) and inserted the first needle. My client was surprised at the lack of discomfort, and I praised her for 'facing her fear'. Next I located and needled Ren 4 (Guanyuan) and without any further fuss I located and needled an Ahshi point 0.3 cun lateral and distal to Ren 12 (Zhongwan) on the right. This point reflected where the pain was coming from around the right eye. The depth of this needle was quite superficial at approximately 0.2 cun. The Ren points ('Heaven and Earth') were fixed to a depth of 0.5 cun for Ren 4 (Guanyuan) and 0.2 or 0.3 cun for Ren 12 (Zhongwan) (see Fig 4.4).

I checked with Mary regarding how she felt. First I enquired if any of the needles were uncomfortable and when she responded that she didn't feel any of them, I highlighted this point and once again praised her for overcoming her fear of needles! Now that she was feeling relaxed I asked her where the pain was. She replied with disbelief that the headache was gone.

Comments

In this case I chose to use Ren 4 (Guanyuan) over Ren 6 (Qihai) for a number of reasons. Mary was very anxious and I felt that using the prescription 'Heaven and Earth' Ren 12 (Zhongwan) and Ren 4 (Guanyuan) would be calming and still move the Stagnant Qi that was causing her headache (See chapter 7, *What's the Point*). This prescription was minimal and powerful and it achieved great results. All the needles were inserted and fixed within about two or three minutes, leaving little time for Mary to get cold feet and change her mind.

At the end of the treatment Mary couldn't believe how much better she felt and she likened it to feeling like floating as she was so relaxed. In this case I was able to help Mary overcome her genuine needle phobia. I was able to show her how effective AA is and emphasise the rapid therapeutic power of this very gentle form of acupuncture. She now has an interesting 'feel good' story to tell her friends at dinner parties, and will be enthusiastic about referring clients!

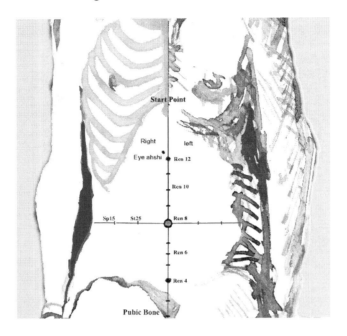

Fig 4.4.Prescription for case history 'Needle Phobic with a Headache'

Ren 3 (Zhongji) 'Middle Extremity'

Functions of Ren 3 (Zhongji)

- Front Mu point of the Bladder;
- Meeting point of the Ren, Liver, Spleen and Kidneys;
- Resolves Damp Heat;
- Improves the Bladders Qi transformation function;
- Clears Heat;

- Is a very important point to treat all genito-urinary (including prostate) problems.

Ren 3 (Zhongji) Abdominal Significance

- It is anatomically equivalent to the coccyx.

Point Location

4 cun inferior to the centre of the umbilicus.

Needling Depths for Different Conditions

This point is rarely used. Depths for this point tend to be shallower as it is at the tail of the turtle. To treat problems with the coccyx the depth will range from 0.3-0.4cun.

Kid 13 (Qixue) 'Qi Hole

Functions of Kid 13 (Qixue) 'Qi Hole'

- Qixue – Qi hole is the meeting point of the Kidney and Penetrating (Chong) Vessel;
- Tonifies the Kidneys Qi and Essence;
- Regulates the Conception (Ren) and Penetrating (Chong) Vessel;
- Regulates the lower Jiao;

- Removes obstruction and masses from the abdomen and chest;
- Treats many menstrual and fertility issues;
- Calms 'running piglet' Qi, eases fear and fright.

Running piglet Qi is experienced as a sensation of energy rushing through the body. Originating from the lower abdomen travelling up the body to the throat and/or the limbs, it can leave the patient feeling close to death and almost paralysed with fear. *'Running piglet disorder arises from the lower abdomen; it rushes up to the throat with such ferocity that the patient feels close to death. It attacks and then remits. It is brought about by fear and fright,'* (Zhang, Z. 2013; Deadman P. et al., 2011).

Kid 13 (Qixue) Abdominal Significance

- Bi-dimensional relationship with the U.B. channel relates to UB 25 (Dachangshu);
- Strong tonification for the Kidneys re-enforces the action of Ren 4 (Guanyuan);
- Often used to reinforce Ren 4 (Guanyuan) and, therefore, nourish the Kidneys to strengthen Bones;
- It has a strong emotional effect of calming fear and fright;
- These points are also frequently used for fertility and all kinds of menstrual problems.

Further Comments and Abdominal Significance

As mentioned these points are equivalent to UB 25 (Dachangshu) and, therefore, can treat lumbar problems more lateral to the spine in the region of L-4. These points are often used to reinforce the effect of Ren 4 (Guanyuan) and thus gives extra tonification to the Kidneys. As a result of the effect on the Kidney energy the connection with the Chong Mai (Conception Vessel) and their anatomical location, Kid 13 (Qixue) points are regularly used in fertility and other aspects of women's health. I often use them for their powerful calming nature for anxious and fearful clients.

Point Location

They are located 0.5 cun either side of Ren 4 (Guanyuan). Note that 0.5 cun is acquired by using the universal 1/2cun measurement from the horizontal measurements (see horizontal measurements by eye chapter 3, *Abdominal Point Location: Get to the Point!).*

Needling Depths for Different Conditions

Needle more superficially 0.1–0.3 or 0.4 cun for more frontal pelvic conditions and more deep for treating the lower back 0.5-0.75 cun. When using these points to enhance the tonification of the Kidneys for fertility or menstrual conditions, the depth can range from 0.5–1.0 cun depending on the weight of the client.

Other Kid points used include 17, 18 and 19. All are connected with the Penetrating Vessel and so these points have a strong calming effect on the Heart and nourish Blood and the Uterus.

Kid 17 (Shangqu) 'Intestine Bend'

Functions of Kid 17 (Shangqu)

- It is used locally to treat abdominal pain;
- It treats the colon, constipation and diarrhoea;
- Removes accumulation.

Kid 17 (Shangqu) Abdominal Significance

- Often used to correct neck pain radiating into the upper back and the shoulders;
- Used contralaterally to open the gate for energy to move to the opposite upper limb when treating problems affecting areas such as the wrist, elbow or fingers;
- Anatomically it is along the medial UB meridian 1.5 cun lateral to the Du Mai at the level of the 7th cervical vertebra;
- It can be used to move Qi into the neck and head for certain types of headaches.

Point Location

Is located 0.5cun lateral to Ren10 (Xiawan).

Needling Depths for Different Conditions

Needle more superficially 0.1 – 0.3 for frontal neck and chest issues, slightly deeper 0.3-0.4 cun for more neck or trapezius conditions and deeper still for treating the upper back 0.4-0.5 cun.

Something to note is that if you wish to activate Huato Jiaji points these will be located between the Ren and the Kidney meridian. Needle depth for stimulating points on the back will usually be at the deeper end of the heaven layer at 0.4-0.5 cun.

Kid 18 (Shiguan) 'Stone Gate'

Functions of Kid 18 (Shiguan)

- Harmonizes the Stomach;
- Regulates the lower Jiao;
- Relieves local pain;
- Regulates the Ren and Chong Vessels.

Kid 18 (Shiguan) Abdominal Significance

- It is often used to strengthen neck muscles and to correct problems in the vicinity of cervical vertebra no. 1 (C-1);
- It treats all kinds of throat problems.

Point Location

Kid 18 is located along the Kidney meridian 0.5 cun lateral to Ren11 (Jianli).

Needling Depths for Different Conditions

Needle superficially 0.1–0.2 for frontal throat conditions and more deep 0.3-0.4 cun for treating the upper neck in the vicinity of GB20 (Feng chi).

Remember that the neck is outside of the turtle's shell and so it is more exposed. Therefore, needle depths are usually not as deep as those points that are within the turtle shell. This also applies to points below Ren 4 (Guanyuan).

Kid 19 (Yindu) 'Yin Metropolis'

Functions of Kid 19 (Yindu)

- Harmonizes the Stomach;
- Regulates the lower Jiao;
- Relieves local pain;
- Regulates the Ren and Chong Mai.

Kid 19 (Yindu) Abdominal Significance

- Can be used to treat head problems as well as reinforcing the action of Ren 12;

- Anatomically these points are in the region of the mouth, in line with St 5 (Daying), and so could be used to treat problems in this area, including stiff and painful jaw due to teeth grinding! (See below, case history 'Discotheque Dislocated Jaw').

Point Location

Kid 19 is located along the Kidney meridian 0.5 cun lateral to Ren 12.

Needling Depths for Different Conditions

Needle depth will be quite superficial at 0.1-0.2 cun for toothache or frontal headache. For headaches at the back of the head, the depth will be 0.3-0.4 cun. For jaw pain, the depth can be anywhere between 0.2-0.3 cun.

CASE STUDY: Discotheque Dislocated Jaw (Facial Pain)

Barry had been in a bar brawl when he was 21, which had resulted in him getting quite a few kicks and punches in the face that dislocated his jaw and fractured his skull.

He decided to try acupuncture at 40 years of age as the pain in his jaw was constant and eating was becoming more difficult. All food had to be bitesize and anything bigger, such as burgers, would result in his jaw dislocating again and making a very audible click. He had pain particularly on the right side of the mandible around the zygomatic arch in the area of

St 7 (Xiaguan) and GB 3 (Shangguan). The pain radiated down to St 5 (Daiyang) and up as far as extra point Taiyang (M-HN-9). The pain and inconvenience were getting progressively worse particularly in the cold winter months.

As Barry was otherwise healthy – though very nervous about needles - it was decided to take as minimal an approach as possible. The prescription used was 'Heaven and Earth' / Sky-Ground, i.e. Ren 12 (Zhongwan) and Ren 4 (Guanyuan). Kidney 19 (Yindu) was punctured quite superficially (0.2-0.3 cun) on the right, enabling me to work on the lower jaw area. Ahshi points approximately 0.3 cun above Kidney 19 (Yindu) were found to have small but obvious nodes that felt quite solid. Three needles were used in a triangular format to give a strong delivery of Qi in the affected area (see fig 4.5). The node was broken up and when asked how the pain was it had decreased by 60%. Treatment was repeated twice that week and bi-weekly for another two weeks. At the end of the six sessions the jaw was much better. The pain had gone. On the occasion when the mouth had opened fully it only clicked a small bit and didn't cause any discomfort. Eighteen months has passed since the end of the treatments, and there is still no pain.

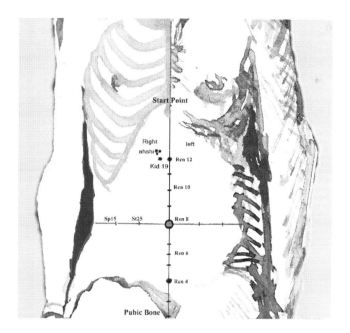

Fig 4.5. AA Prescription for case 'Discotheque Dislocated Jaw'

Stomach 24 (Huaroumen) 'Slippery Flesh Gate'

Functions of Stomach 24 (Huaroumen)

- Transforms Phlegm and calms the spirit;
- Harmonises the Stomach and stops vomiting;
- Stops vomiting with Blood and treats mania depression.

Stomach 24 (Huaroumen) Abdominal Significance

- St 24 (Huaroumen) anatomically is equivalent to the shoulder;

- This point is important to strengthen the upper back muscles such as the rhomboideus minor and major, the levator scapulae and the trapezius;
- Eases spasm in the above muscle groups and stops pain in the upper back;
- The Stomach Yangming meridian is in charge of flesh and has abundant Blood and Qi, therefore the St 24 (Huaroumen) distributes Qi and Blood to the upper extremities and the head.

St 24 (Huaroumen) and points 0.2 cun inferior and medial can also be used to treat sinusitis or hay fever. This is because these points are anatomically equivalent to point Lung 1 (Zhongfu).

Point Location

St 24 (Huaroumen) is located 1 cun directly above St 25 (Tianshu) on a line level with Ren 9 (Shuifen).

Needling Depths for Different Conditions

When treating shoulder problems affecting the front, needles are inserted to a depth ranging from 0.1-0.3 cun. When treating the back of the shoulder needles need to be deeper at 0.3-0.5 cun. If the problem is acute, needles should be shallower than if the condition is chronic. To treat the upper back, the depth should be 0.3-0.5 cun. If the problem is with the skin, the needles will often be at a depth of 0.1 cun or less, i.e. very superficial!

Stomach 25 (Tianshu), 'Heavenly Pillar'

Functions of St 25 (Tianshu)

- Promotes the function of the Large Intestine (LI);
- Front Mu of the LI;
- Clears Heat from the Stomach and Intestines;
- Regulates the Stomach and Spleen;
- Regulates Qi;
- Is especially good for treating Excess conditions of the Stomach.

St 25 (Tianshu) Abdominal Significance

- Also used to clear (any) Heat through LI;
- Used to clear Dampness through the LI:
- Used for back problems (centre) treats large muscles (latissimus dorsi) of the back;
- In conjunction with St 24 (Huaroumen) and 26 (Wailing) can remove muscle spasm throughout the back.

Because of its relationship with the LI it treats the Lung (See Baqua) and is especially useful for treating coughs and asthma. This is because the front Mu pt. of the LI it is capable of regulating the 3 Jiao's upper via Lungs, its paired organ, middle Jiao through the St, its associated organ, and the lower Jiao by virtue of its anatomical location and function (Lore, R. 2011).

Point Location

St 25 (Tianshu) is located by dividing the area from the centre of the belly button to the outer limit of the side in 3 it is at the border of the 1st $1/3^{rd}$ i.e. 2 cun lateral to the centre of Ren 8 (Shenque).

Needling Depths for Different Conditions

St 25 (Tianshu) is one of the most frequently used points. When using it to treat mid-back problems, it is needled to a depth of 0.3-0.5 cun or deeper if the patient is larger. When using it to clear Heat through the LI, it is needled slightly deeper to a level of 0.4-0.7cun. To treat asthma and coughs, it is needled to a similar depth. When needling St 25 (Tianshu) to treat the Lung through the Ba Gua hologram, it should be needled to a depth greater than 1 cun in the Gua of Dui on the left.

Stomach 26 (Wailing) 'Outer Mound'

Functions of St 26 (Wailing)

- Regulates Qi and alleviates pain;
- Indicated for severe abdominal pain;
- Useful point to treat hernia
- Treats all kinds of Shan* disorder;

- Dysmenorrhoea/amenorrhoea.

*Shan disorder is a TCM term that incorporates a number of possible conditions including hernia, external genital swelling and other complications due to Stagnation of Qi such as constipation and incomplete or difficult urination (Shan Disorder TCM Term, n.d).

St 26 (Wailing) Abdominal Significance

- Anatomically it relates to the hip (turtle hologram);
- Strengthens the lower back;
- Relieves pain and spasm in the lower back muscles including the quadratus lumborum, longissimus and gluteus minimus, middimis and maximus. It has this effect whether the condition is chronic or acute;
- St 26 (Wailing) distributes Qi and Blood to the lower extremities.

Point Location

St 26 (Wailing) is located 1 cun inferior to St 25 (Tianshu) on a horizontal line with Ren 7 (Yinjiao). Note the 1 cun measurement below the umbilicus can be very different to the 1 cun measurement above.

Needling Depths for Different Conditions

When treating hip problems affecting the front, needles are inserted to depths ranging from 0.1-0.3 cun depending on where the pain is located. When treating the back of the hip needles need to be deeper at 0.3-0.5 cun. If the problem is acute needles should be shallower than if the condition is chronic. To treat the lower back, the depth should be 0.3-0.5 cun. If the problem is with the skin, the needles will often be at a depth of 0.1 cun or less, i.e. very superficial!

Stomach 27 (Daju) 'Great Gigantic'

Functions of Stomach 27 (Daju)

- Eases abdominal pain due to Excess Stomach conditions;
- Moves Stagnant Qi in the lower abdomen;
- It is often used for treating hernia and male genital problems;
- Dysuria;
- St 27 (Daju) benefits and firms the Essence, regulates Qi and promotes urination.

Stomach 27 (Daju) Abdominal Significance

- Stomach 27 (Daju) is important in abdominal acupuncture for invigorating Qi especially when energy levels are low;
- Anatomically it is equivalent to Kid 1 (Yongquan);
- It can treat neuralgia of the feet and it is particularly effective when this is due to diabetes.

Point Location

It is located 1 cun inferior to St 26 (Wailing).

Needling Depths for Different Conditions

When using this point to invigorate Qi it should be needled to a depth of 0.8-0.9 cun. If treating feet problems, usually superficial needling to a depth of between 0.2-0.3 cun is sufficient. (See case histories, 'Diabetic Feet', 'Twinkle Toes that had lost their Sparkle' and 'The Fabulous Flipper Foot', in chapter 8, *Abdominal Acupuncture Prescriptions for Frequently Seen Painful Conditions.*).

Spleen 15 (Daheng) 'Great Horizontal'

Functions of Spleen 15 (Daheng)

- Strengthens the Spleen;
- Nourishes the limbs;
- Resolves Damp;
- Moves Qi and regulates the intestines;
- Stops pain;
- It is particularly good for treating any Excess condition of the abdomen.

Abdominal Significance Sp 15 (Daheng)

- Indications: Important point to treat (Deficiency) chronic constipation;
- Diarrhea with mucus in stool and Dampness;
- This is the outermost point of abdominal acupuncture;

- It is good for nourishing muscles;
- Tonifies the Spleen;
- Expels Damp from muscles and joints;
- Sp 15 (Daheng) on the left is used to treat the lower Jiao at the earth level (Ba Qua).

This is the outermost point of the Ba Gua and acts on the flanks. This point is also used to resolve pain from the muscles and joints, especially when due to Dampness. Additionally, it is used to stop lower back pain and resolve back spasm. It is also useful to use for chronic back pain as it will help to nourish muscles that have been weakened as a result.

Point Location

Spleen 15 (Daheng) is located in the same way as with regular acupuncture at the lateral border of the rectus abdominis muscle level with the umbilicus. It is 4 cun from the centre of the umbilicus or two-thirds (2/3's) the way from the umbilicus to the outer flank (Fig 4.1).

Needling Depths for Different Conditions

Sp 15 (Daheng) is needled to a depth of approximately 0.5 - 0.75 cun in order to treat lower back pain. When treating pain around the lateral border of the body level with the umbilicus, for example, rib pain, the depth should be more superficial between 0.1 and 0.3 cun.

Functions of special abdominal acupuncture points

Ab 1 (elbow)

Is also known as arthritic point 1 or upper rheumatism point

This point is multi-functional:

- Anatomically it relates to the elbow;
- It is used to clear Wind Damp and, therefore, it treats Bi Syndrome;
- On the left side it is used to treat Spleen Qi problems. This can be explained by the fact that it is located in the Kūn Gua when using the Ba Gua hologram. The Kūn Gua represents the Spleen. This point is also known as Shang Fen Xi which indicates its potency for clearing Wind Damp;
- On the right side it is used to treat Liver Qi problems due to the fact that it is located in the Xun Gua of the Ba Gua. This point can also be used to treat other problems of the middle Jiao.

Point Location

Ab1 (Elbow) is located a half cun superior to and a 1/2 cun lateral to St 24 (Huaroumen) the shoulder point (Fig 4.1).

Needling Depths for Different Conditions

When treating skin conditions on the elbow area, the depth of the needle is very superficial at 0.1 cun or less. Treating elbow problems depends on the location of the problem. Upper elbow will be more superficial at between 0.1-0.2 cun while pain at the back of the elbow will need to be needled between 0.2-0.4 cun. When using Ab 1 point to treat Wind Damp or Sp/Liver Qi, the depth should be 0.5 cun or more.

Ab 2 Wrist Point

Ab 2 (wrist) is known as arthritic point 2 or upper lateral rheumatism point.

- Ab 2 anatomically relates to the wrist on the turtle hologram;
- It also helps to clear Wind Damp and is used to treat Bi Syndrome.

Note the terms rheumatism and arthritic points are often interchanged, and I have seen them referred to as both of these. I was taught the term 'rheumatism points' in China and so that is the term I favour. When these points are used collectively in the form of 'Feng Shi Dian' to treat Bi Syndrome with Wind and Dampness they are referred to as Upper Rheum (Ab 1) or upper Lateral Rheum (Ab 2) etc.

Point Location

(Ab 2) wrist points are a ½ cun lateral and a half cun inferior to elbow points, so that the shoulder, elbow and wrist look like an inverted **V** (Fig 4.1).

Needling Depths for Different Conditions

When treating skin conditions on the wrist area, the depth of the needle is very superficial at 0.1 cun or less. Treating wrist problems the depths are usually quite superficial so use your client's feedback to inform you what depth works. When using Ab 2 point to treat Wind Damp, the depth should be 0.5 cun or more.

Ab3 (Arthritic 3)

- Anatomically it relates to the thumb.

Point Location

Ab 3 is located 1cun directly superior to Ab 2 (see Fig 4.1).

Needling Depths for Different Conditions

Thumb problems require superficial needle depths of approximately 0.1-0.2 cun or less (See Fig 4.1).

Ab4 Arthritic 4 or lower rheumatism point/ knee point

- Anatomically it relates to the knee;

- It is used to clear Wind Damp. The pinyin name for this point is Xia Fen Shi and it treats Bi Syndrome;

- Ab 4 on the right resides in the Gen Gua of the Ba Gua and it dominates the upper Jiao and, therefore, treats problems in this area also.

Point Location

Ab 4 knee point is a half cun inferior and a ½ cun lateral to St 26 (Wailing) the hip point (Fig. 4.1).

Needling Depths for Different Conditions

When treating skin conditions on the knee area, the depth of the needle is very superficial at 0.1 cun or less. Treating knee problems depends on the location of the problem frontal knee will be more superficial at between 0.1-0.3 cun. Pain at the back of the knee will need to be needled between 0.2-0.4 cun. When using Ab 4 point to treat Wind Damp of the lower limbs, the depth should be 0.5 cun or more.

Ab 5 Arthritic 5 medial knee pt.

- Anatomically it relates to the medial knee.

Point Location

Ab 5 medial knee point is 1 cun medial to Ab 4, with the knee on a line level with Ren 6 (Qihai) point. As mentioned before, points are fluid and therefore when treating problems of the medial knee feel for the Ahshi point. It may be halfway between Ab 4 and Ab 5 (See Fig 4.1).

Needling Depths for Different Conditions

When treating skin conditions on the knee area, the depth of the needle is very superficial at 0.1 cun or less. Treating medial knee problems the depth normally will be between 0.1-0.3 cun.

Ab 6 Ankle point arthritic 6 or lower lateral rheumatism point

- Ab 6 is known as ankle or arthritic point 6;
- Ab 6 anatomically relates to the ankle;
- It also helps to clear Wind Damp and Bi Syndrome.

Point Location

Ab 6, the ankle point, is on a line ½ cun lateral and a half cun inferior to the knee point. Hip, knee and ankle should look like a backslash \ (see Fig 4.1).

Needling Depths for Different Conditions

When treating skin conditions on the ankle area, the depth of the needle is very superficial at 0.1cun or less. Treating ankle problems depends on the location of the problem but, as it is quite superficial, it is best to get feedback from your client as to what depth ameliorates the pain. When using the ankle point (Ab 6) to treat Wind Damp, the depth should be 0.5cun or more.

Ab 7 Qipang

This point is used to direct Qi from the Kidneys down through the opposite hip, knee and ankle. It is also used for lower back pain in the vicinity of vertebra L1-2. It is where the sacrum begins.

Point Location

Qipang (Ab 7) is located ½ cun lateral to Ren 6 along the Kidney meridian (see Fig 4.1).

Needling Depths for Different Conditions

This point is usually used to treat back pain and so it is needled to a depth of 0.5 cun or deeper.

Ab 8 Qi Wai

This point is used to treat irregular and painful menstruation. It also treats abdominal pain and digestive disorders.

Point Location

1 cun lateral to Ren 6.

Needling Depths for Different Conditions

When using this point for menstrual problems the depth will be between 1.0 and 1.5 cun.

Abdominal Ba Gua Acupuncture.

(Indications from various sources, including Dr. Han Yan Personal communication 2005, and Yang. C. 2012)

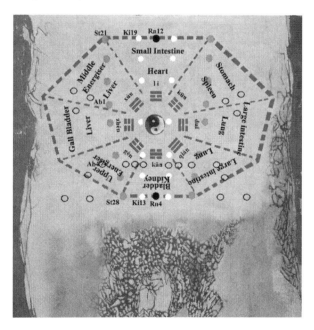

Fig 4.6. The Ba Gua map used in AA at the earth level

Li Trigram (fire) Ht / SI

Treats insomnia, palpitations, excessive and vivid dreams, forgetfulness, poor concentration, and dementia. It also treats digestive and absorption disorders.

Using Point Ren 12 Zhongwan.

Kun Trigram (Earth) Sp / St

Qi and Blood Deficiency patterns, Sp treats lack of appetite, diarrhoea, easy to bruise, abdominal distension, bloating and loose stool.

Using Point Left Elbow point (Ab1).

Dui Trigram (Lake) Lu / Li

The lower Jiao is treated through the Dui Gua.

Using Point Sp 15 (Daheng) on the left.

Qian Trigram (Heaven) Lu / Li

Treats asthma, cough, fullness in the chest, diarrhea and constipation.

Using Point Left Ab 4 (knee) point.

Kăn Trigram (Water) Kid / UB

Treats weak knees, lower back ache, dysuria, incontinence, frequent urination, oedema and low libido.

Using Point Ren 4 (Guanyuan).

Gen Trigram (Mountain) Upper Jiao

Problems of the upper Jiao, Lung and Wei Qi Deficiency leading to recurrent colds, etc.

Using Point right Ab 4 (knee) point.

Zhen Trigram (Thunder) Liv /GB

Treats Liver and Gallbladder disorders (see Xun below)

Using Point Sp 15 (Daheng) on the right.

Xun Trigram (Wind) Liv and Middle Jiao

Treats hypochondriac pain, PMT, dysmenorrhoea, irregular menses, tinnitus, vertigo, fullness in the chest, indigestion, reflux, loose stools, constipation, blurred vision muscles cramps, etc.

Treats the middle Jiao and Liver Qi problems.

Using Point Right elbow point Ab 1

See Appendix Table A1 for Quick Reference Chart highlighting AA Ren points.

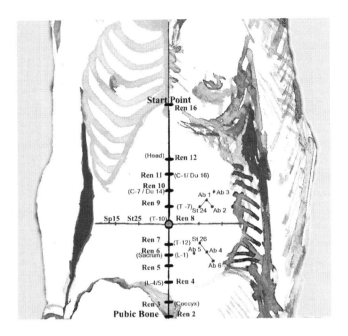

Start Point
Ren 16

(Head) Ren 12

Ren 11 (C-1/ Du 16)
Ren 10
(C-7 / Du 14)
Ren 9
(T -7) St 24 Ab 1 Ab 3
Ab 2
Sp15 St25 (T-10) Ren 8

Ren 7
(T-12) St 26
Ren 6
(Sacrum) (L-1) Ab 5 Ab 4
Ren 5 Ab 6

(L-4/5) Ren 4

Ren 3 (Coccyx)
Pubic Bone Ren 2

Fig. 4.7 Anatomical importance of main AA points & limb patterns

Summary of Topics Covered in this Chapter

- A detailed look at each of the traditional acupuncture points used in AA including those on the Ren, Kidney, Stomach and Spleen meridians

- Examination of relevant points and a look at each one's abdominal significance as well as the traditional functions and special energetic importance of particular points

- Discussion of each of the eight unique abdominal (Ab) points concerning anatomical relevance and functions

- Needle depths were described for common ailments relating to each of these points

- Brief description of the AA zones of the Ba Gua.

Chapter 5: Abdominal Diagnosis – Feel the Force

Learning Objectives

In this chapter we will look at the importance of abdominal diagnosis. We will examine how to integrate all the information available from the abdomen into your treatment plan so that you can provide the best possible treatment for your patients. You will learn how to locate and treat Ahshi points with confidence, which will enable you to be more assertive and focused when treating painful conditions. Ahshi points may be a small node or nodule that is not necessarily very painful to touch, but because of the location with respect to the anatomical area being reflected, will cure the painful part of the body being treated with AA.

General Considerations

The abdomen can be used to give other vital clues as to what or where the underlying problem is. Abdominal diagnosis has always played a very important part in ascertaining the overall condition. In ancient times the abdomen was used more for diagnosis and, in fact, in the book, *The Nan Jing*, it states in chapter 7 that the abdomen is more diagnostically relevant than the pulse. In many parts of China palpation became less popular due to social taboos and so over time other diagnostic methods took precedence.

At some stage during the Jin-Yuan dynasty abdominal palpation and other diagnostic techniques, such as channel palpation, lost favour as it was thought to be invasive and disrespectful to touch women, especially women of high social standing such as the emperor's wife (Wang, J, 2013). Indeed, some TCM doctors used a silk thread with one end wrapped around the wrist of the royal lady so that the practitioner could read the pulse from the ulnar artery simply by holding the other end of the silk thread. Needles were also often inserted through clothing to avoid touching someone as significant at the emperor's wife. (Reid, T. 2008).

The Japanese continued to use abdominal or *Hara* diagnosis in therapies such as Japanese meridian acupuncture and Shiatsu. Some of the zones used in some Japanese *Hara* diagnosis systems are similar to those used in abdominal acupuncture.

Diagnosis using the abdomen requires a sensitivity that takes practice to cultivate. Always use gentle force and focus on what you feel.

As discussed earlier in chapter 2, *What Makes Abdominal So Phenomenal!* the abdomen has many energetically important points including front Mu points. On palpation these points and different areas of the abdomen may indicate Qi Stagnation, Blood Stasis, Phlegm, Deficiency or Excess in the relevant organs or anatomically related area (depending on the depth of the irregularities). You can see this reflected by the hologram of the turtle (Fig 5.1) or the abdominal Ba Gua (Fig 5.2).

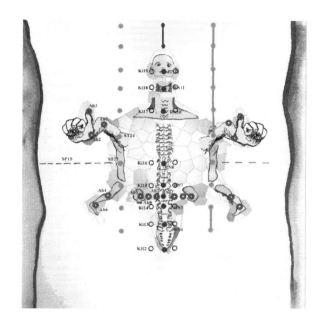

Fig 5.1. Abdominal acupuncture chart of the turtle

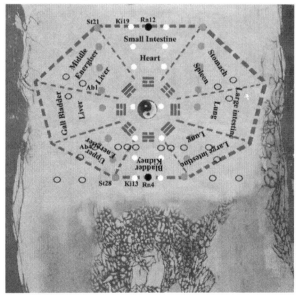

Fig 5.2. The abdominal Ba Gua chart

~ 155 ~

Since the umbilicus is in the centre of the abdomen, and as Ren 8 (Shenque) is the origin of the AMS and the Jing Lou meridian systems, the umbilicus and its surrounding area can give a lot of pertinent diagnostic information.

In my practice, I always try and maintain a certain dignity and respect for my client. Exposing a client's midriff can be embarrassing for some and it can make some people feel a little vulnerable. In situations like this it is important to communicate what you are doing and re- assure your patient.

> **Tip:** Warm your hands before putting them on a person's abdomen, and be gentle. Start with a very light touch and gradually depress more firmly if necessary. It is kind of like cooking - it's better to add strong ingredients slowly. So get feedback and increase if necessary. A gentle touch ensures subtle information being transmitted through the pads of your fingers while being too heavy can result in slight discrepancies and vital information being missed.

Reasons why the Abdomen is so important from the ancient book the Nan Jing

The abdomen is the site of:

- Origin of vital (Qi);
- (And of) the Triple Burner, which distributes all Ying and Wei (Qi);
- Foundation of all 12 (channels);
- (And) of the (Zang Fu);

- Gate of the breath;
- 'Spirit guarding against evil';
- A person's root and foundation (Lore, R. 2005).

Overview of the Abdomen

Observe the overall abdominal picture including colour, temperature, the muscle tone and the shape of the navel. Note the distance between Ren 12 (Zhongwan) and Ren 8 (Shenque) and from the umbilicus to Ren 4 (Guanyuan). A relatively longer distance from the Umbilicus to the top of the Pubic bone indicates a strong constitutional life force and Essence than a shorter distance.

Look for any moles or discolouration and take note of where they are with relevance to what meridian they are on. These may indicate Heat, Stasis or Cold. Observe any scars, they should never be needled directly but can be needled on either side. Scars can result in a blockage of the flow of Qi and Blood in the related meridian. Nodes or nodules can indicate Qi or Blood Stagnation. These may indicate Ahshi points relating to the relevant anatomical area of the body where there is a problem.

The abdomen of a man should be firmer than that of a woman since men are more Yang in nature. A flaccid Stomach on a man often indicates Yang Deficiency.

Hair is a manifestation of the Ren and relates to Yin and Blood. Hair below the navel on a woman indicates Kidney Yin Deficiency and often implies the presence of menstrual problems such as endometriosis. Check acupuncture point Kid 3 (Tai Qi). If it forms a large depression, this confirms this diagnosis. (Dr. Han Yan, 2002, personal communication).

Diagnosis through Palpation of the Umbilicus

Dr. Yu Geng Chu emphasises the importance of palpating the umbilicus in diagnosis. The umbilicus is at the centre of the abdomen and the transfer of Jing, Shen, Qi and Blood, and it has a close relationship with the Ren Mai (Bo. Z, 1993, pp. 13-14).

- If the umbilicus feels tough in the upper and lower abdomen it indicates Deficiency of the Spleen and Kidney;
- When the patient feels distension around the umbilicus it shows disharmony of the Spleen and the Kidney;
- Should the patient feel a throbbing sensation from the upper part of the umbilicus this indicates disharmony between the Heart and Liver;
- If there is detectable and palpable Qi in the upper part of the belly button, this indicates Deficiency Cold in the lower Jiao. This is because the Deficient Kidney Yang is floating as a result of the patient's Empty Cold of the Spleen and Kidney. If the palpable Qi is on the left or the right, it suggests disharmony of the Liver and Gallbladder.

Shape and Quality of the Umbilicus

- A normal navel is round and deep with creases in the surrounding walls which indicate strong Kidney and Spleen Qi and plenty of energy;

- An umbilicus that is convex and protrudes outwards indicates weak Spleen and Kidneys. The umbilicus should have strong tendons to pull it in;
- A long narrow shape to the navel indicates Kidney Vacuity;
- A small flabby belly button reveals weak Spleen Qi;
- A triangular shape to the navel indicates digestive problems due to the Liver overacting on the Spleen;
- A longer distance between the umbilicus and Ren 4 (Guanyuan) indicates good vital Qi.

Temperature

Feel the temperature above and below your client's umbilicus using the back of your hand. The back of the hand will be more sensitive to subtle temperature changes. Feel the temperature around Ren 8 (Shenque) and in each of the main areas of the Baqua (see Figs 5.1 and 5.2).

The depth of temperature variation indicates area or level (heaven, humanity or earth) affected.

- Cold temperature indicates Yang or Qi Xu in the relevant anatomical area (as seen on the map of the turtle) or the organ represented by the Bagua chart;
- Cold temperature in the left elbow position (Ab 2) may indicate a tennis elbow or, if the Cold seems to be coming from a deeper level, it may indicate a Spleen Qi Vacuity. Similarly, Cold around the shoulder St 24 (Huaroumen area may indicate frozen shoulder;

- Look for Heat spots or local warmth that may suggest Excess Heat, invasion of Heat or Yin Vacuity. The depth of the Heat will again highlight whether it is an anatomical or Zang Fu issue;
- Cold above and below the navel indicates Spleen and Kidney Yang Deficiency and has a poor prognosis (unless it is due to environmental temperature);
- Cold above the umbilicus indicates Sp Yang / Qi Def;
- Excessive Heat around Ren 12 (Zhongwan) may indicate herpes zoster attacking the head and face area. It may also suggest a toothache or abscess if more superficial.

Colour

Check the colour of the whole abdomen. Look for any colour changes and note the areas that these may occur. As with the temperature above, the area, depth and intensity will help with the diagnosis.

- Dark colour around Ren 4 (Guanyuan) indicates Yang Deficiency;
- Red spots show Heat in the related area.

Nodes / Nodules / Ahshi Points

Nodes and nodules may be felt as subtle hair like accumulations or they may be the size of a grain of rice or even as big as a pea.

Nodes are due to:

- Blood Stagnation;

- Phlegm accumulation or a combination of this with Blood Stagnation;
- Nodes at Ren 9 (Shuifen) indicate Damp;
- Nodes felt at superficial (Heaven) level indicates Ahshi point of related part of the body, e.g. hip, shoulder, vertebra, etc.

If nodules are felt either side of the umbilicus this indicates Spleen Dampness. Nodes below Ren 8 (Shenque), however, indicates Stagnation or Damp Heat in the lower Jiao. Moving down towards Ren 4 (Guanyuan) the presence of these accumulations can indicate Damp Heat in the lower Jiao affecting the Urinary Bladder in the form of a urinary tract infection (UTI). They may also indicate vertebra problems represented by an Ahshi point and should be needled through the resistance and even broken down by some needle manipulations such as vigorous rotations. This should result in the pain reducing substantially.

Nodes at Sp Qi point (left elbow Ab 1) indicate the presence of internal Damp. If they are shallow, they suggest elbow pain, though if they are deep with loose and dry stool or constipation they suggest Spleen Vacuity. If they are found at a deep level on the right elbow point (Ab 1), this suggests Liver and/or Gall Bladder problems.

Be patient, open and intuitive when palpating. First, get a general sense and then zone into where you expect there to be some discrepancy. Once located in the area expected nodes or nodules will often be the Ahshi point that relieves pain. Don't miss it by being unaware, impatient or too heavy-handed.

> **Tip:** When assessing the abdomen of larger clients you may find the presence of many nodes or nodules which indicates Phlegm accumulation. Be selective when looking for specific Ahshi points to resolve pain in a particular area. If the node or nodule is in the anatomical area (as represented by the turtle) that you are addressing then select that node, needle it and get feedback so that you can eliminate the correct point to use rapidly.

CASE STUDY: Norman's Neuralgia (Nerve Pain following Shingles)

Norman suffered a severe case of herpes zoster (shingles) which affected him at the end of the coccyx around Du 1 (Changqiang) and Ren 1(Huiyin). He came to the clinic three weeks after the shingles had cleared up with paroxysmal pain and itching in the surrounding area. The bouts of pain were at times unbearable, and the itch resulted in scratching until the area bled.

Observation of the abdomen revealed Heat in the area of Ren 3 (Zhongji) to Ren 4 (Guanyuan) with some fine nodules in this area the size of a half grain of rice. The aim of the treatment was to stop pain, clear Heat and Dampness in the lower Jiao and restore normal function to the Ren, Du and Urinary Bladder meridians.

The prescription used was Ren 12 (Zhongwan) Ren 10 (Xiawan) Ren 4 (Guanyuan). The area between Ren 3 (Zhongji) and 4 (Guanyuan) where the nodes were felt was needled to a depth of only 0.3 cun. This was deep enough to dissolve the blockages and relieve pain due to its anatomical relationship with the coccyx. This area is often needled to a lesser depth due to the fact that it is at the tail of the turtle (and therefore is more exposed). St 25 (Tianshu) was used to help to clear Excess Damp Heat through the Large Intestine. Meanwhile Ren 10 (Xiawan) was needled slightly inferiorly to act on Du 14 (Dahzui) and assist in clearing Heat. The right elbow point Ab 1 was used to harmonise the Liver and Gall Bladder while the left knee area Ab 4 was used to expel Dampness through the lower Jiao (see Fig 5.3).

Norman's pain and itchy irritation had improved by 60% by the second session, and abdominal acupuncture continued to be the main treatment protocol. After the third visit episodes of discomfort and itch were rare and when they did occur they were mild and only lasted for a short time. On his next appointment, Norman revealed that the pain had returned for about 30 minutes on the previous night after he had consumed a lot of alcohol. I explained that alcohol (also known as 'Fire water' in Chinese medicine) is hot and that this exacerbated the Damp Heat nature of the neuralgia. This was the reason his pain and irritating itch had returned!

The next three sessions saw the problem disappear, and it has not returned since. Neuralgia after shingles can be very persistent and last up to 18 months. In Norman's case, the problem was completely resolved after eight treatments.

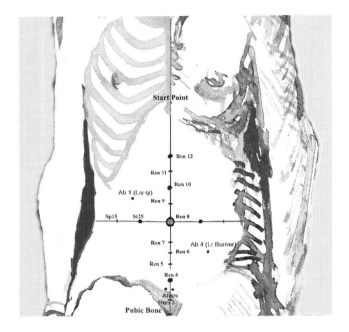

Start Point

Ren 12
Ren 11
Ren 10
Ab 1 (Liv qi)
Ren 9
Sp15   St25   Ren 8
Ren 7   Ab 4 (Lr Burner)
Ren 6
Ren 5
Ren 4
Ahshi
Ren 3
Pubic Bone

Fig 5.3. AA Prescriptions for case history 'Normans Neuralgia'

Summary of Topics Covered in this Chapter

The abdomen needs to be looked at and examined with all aspects considered including:

- Overall appearance
- Navel shape and depth
- General and localised colour
- Tense or flaccid abdomen on palpation
- Temperature, general and localised
- Presence and position of nodes or nodules
- Location of Ahshi points.

Chapter 6: Abdominal Acupuncture Treatment Protocols

Learning Objectives

This chapter details all aspects of AA treatment protocols. I will discuss how to receive and interpret the subtle messages from the needles and what response to this information will give the best treatment result. This is a natural progression from the diagnosis described in chapter 5, and the subtle cues ascertained from each needle used will often offer confirmation of your initial conclusions while giving more insight into the specifics of each case. You will also learn needle manipulations to use so that abdominal acupuncture works at its optimum for you and your clients.

General Considerations

Be aware of the potential contra-indications when using AA as listed below.

Contra–Indications

- Pregnancy;
- Enlarged Liver or Spleen;
- Cancer in the area Stomach, Pancreas / Liver;
- Peritonitis;
- Scars - If there are scars needle either side of them *;
- Venous dilation around the navel;
- Acute unexplained abdominal pain.

* Where there are scars, for example along the Ren meridian between Ren 6 (Qihai) and Ren 4 (Guanyuan) simply insert needles approximately 0.2cun lateral to the scar on each side.

As with any acupuncture treatment hygiene is paramount. Hands should be thoroughly washed before each treatment. The area to be needled should be sterilised. I prefer to use iodine 0.75% (though it is becoming more difficult to buy) or *Betadine*. Both of these highlight the locations of the points and emphasise the relevant patterns and landmarks produced by the hologram of the turtle.

Use a Q-tip or a cotton bud to apply the iodine or *Betadine* as it gives better accuracy when locating points over a cotton wool ball. The Q-tip can double up as a ruler for finding and measuring (by eye) the small distance of the **'Universal ½ cun'**. (See chapter 3, *Abdominal Point Location: Get to the Point*).

Use needles ranging in gauge size from 0.16 mm – 0.30 mm preferably abdominal acupuncture needles 25 mm or 40 mm in length, either tubed or un-tubed. I prefer to use 0.22mm or 0.25mm gauge un-tubed needles as freehand gives more subtle information as to any resistance to the needle and the initial insertion can be kept to a more superficial level. The exact point of insertion is likely to be more accurate also when using un-tubed needles.

Position yourself in a comfortably grounded manner at whichever side of your client that feels best for you. I prefer to stand on the left of the client with their head towards my right-hand side. Your eye line should be centred directly above your client's navel. As you observe the abdomen, breathe into your Dantian and settle your mind. Bring your intention to each stage of the treatment, starting with the overall abdominal observation and diagnosis (see chapter 5, *Abdominal Diagnosis: Feel the Force*).

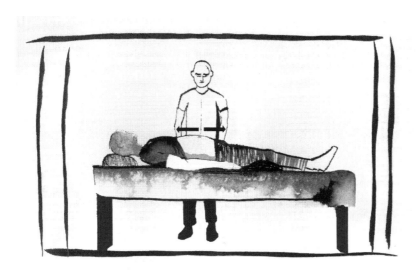

Fig 6.1. Ideal position of practitioner & client for AA observation and treatment

When you have formulated a prescription that will best address your client's problem/s using chapter 7, Prescriptions: *What's the Point?* and chapter 8, *Abdominal Acupuncture Prescriptions for Frequently seen Painful Conditions*, you can then measure and locate the main points (see chapter 3, *Abdominal Point Location: Get to the Point!)* that you will be using in your treatment.

Following this, survey the areas you might expect to feel Ahshi points. Remember that clients with a heavier set will often have many nodes around their abdomen, so be selective and choose nodes in the area of interest only these will be the Ahshi points you want. Make a mental note at first, rather than marking these as you don't want to confuse the picture with lots of potential point markings. (See the tapestry in chapter 9, *Putting it all Together*).

Referencing your Client's Pain or Discomfort

Ask your client to bring their awareness to the pain or discomfort they have in each part of their body as it is **at that very moment**. If they are not in pain when they arrive but have a stiffness or discomfort, ask them to tune into that.

Your client should then score that discomfort or pain in each area at a **reference level of 10 out of 10** or 100% of what that level of discomfort is, **at that very moment in time.** This point is important. Even if the pain is only at a score of 4 out of 10 compared to the previous day, then that subjective 4 is equal to 100% of today's pain, and, therefore, it should be brought up to a score of 10 on the 1-10 reference scale now*. This is often difficult to explain to clients and it is vital to get this concept through to your patient so that they can see the real changes as they occur.

Sometimes it is necessary to palpate the painful area following the insertion and fixing of the needles to accurately gauge the change in the pain levels. If your client finds it difficult to vocalise the difference in pain you can use other cues such as facial expressions. I recently had a client with Down's syndrome and he found it difficult to communicate changes in pain. I found palpating the painful area and observing his expressions gave me all the information I needed.

*An improvement of 30% on a scale of 10 is easier to visualise than an improvement of 30% on a starting pain references score of 4!

> **Tip:** I usually ask clients not to take painkillers before they come for treatment if they can avoid using them. This will impress upon your client the real potential power of AA. When there is a significant decrease in the pain following needling, there will be no question that the pain reduction is due to the AA rather than medication, which, if they've taken something, may just begin to take effect at the very moment that you check what the pain levels are!

The Needle Sequence for Abdominal Acupuncture

- Start from top to bottom on the vertical line such as with the prescription 'Guiding Qi Home' or Sky–Ground (see chapter 7, *Prescriptions: What's the Point?*);
- Then needle from inside to outside on the horizontal line e.g. St 25 (Tianshu) then Sp 15 (Daheng);
- Place needles in the relevant equivalent anatomical area of pain using the hologram of the turtle as a guide, e.g. the hip point St 26 (Wailing). If there are Ahshi points mark them for later when you may need to refine your treatment to cure the pain;
- Insert all the main needles that you are using in the treatment and leave them at a very superficial depth just through the epidermis

before setting them at the required depth. Usually, this is done a couple of minutes after inserting all the needles (see below).

If any of the needles sting it may be because they have hit a capillary, sensory nerve or sweat pore. If it is still painful after a few moments, simply remove the needle, rub the area and reinsert it very close to where it was. Do not reinsert exactly in the same place as this will only cause your client further pain. This is really the only time that abdominal acupuncture is painful although points around Ren 4 (Guanyuan) and Ren 9 (Shuifen) are more likely than other AA points to be painful.

Notes on Needle Depths

Here are some simple rules to remember which will help you to find the right needle depths:

- Shallower needle depth for new and acute conditions, sense organs and anatomical or peripheral limb problems;
- Needles should be deeper for old or chronic conditions, the back of the body and Zang Fu (organ) problems;
- For more specific depths see chapter 7, *Prescriptions: What's the Point?*

Let the Needle Slide and it will be your Guide

When all the main needles are in situ, go back to the first point and start the process of fine tuning. This involves fixing each needle to the correct depth using the following steps to ensure that each one is in the ultimate position to achieve the best possible therapeutic results.

Loosely hold the handle of the needle between your thumb and forefinger. Slide the thumb and forefinger gently down the handle with minimal pressure or force. You will normally have to repeat this sliding technique until the needle naturally stops (see Diagram 6.2) at the correct depth.

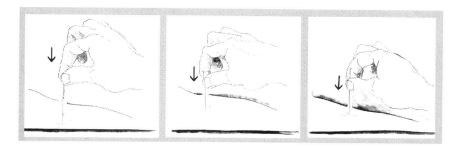

Fig 6.2. AA sliding needle technique

This sliding technique has a very important but subtle difference in abdominal acupuncture when compared to traditional acupuncture needling. This is due to the diagnostic information ascertained through the needle and the different depths that the therapeutic action is focused at when using AA. When doing traditional acupuncture, I don't use this technique as I usually know at what depth I will get to the acupuncture point and the arrival of De-Qi (big fish).

Avoid the temptation to spin or twist the handle as it moves deeper. As your finger and thumb gently slide down the handle of the needle bring your awareness to the way the needle is passing through the different layers of the abdomen. If the needle passes through to the desired depth like it is going through butter this is a sign that there is no major problem in this area. Maintain your focus and position the main prescription points such as 'Guiding Qi Home' to their correct depth. Await the arrival of De-Qi in the form of a slight tugging or gripping of the needle.

The arrival of De-Qi when doing regular acupuncture points was always described in China as being like catching a fish on a hook as the practitioner would feel the arrival of Qi as something like a little pull on the needle. With AA, the arrival of Qi is usually minimal, and so it might feel like a very small fish caught on a hook (it is very subtle)!

With abdominal acupuncture, the clients awareness of De-Qi is much less obvious than with traditional acupuncture points such as LI 4 (Hegu) where the arrival of Qi or de-Qi is quite obvious.

Next it is time to fix the needles at each of the points. This is where the depth is more dependent on the location and the nature of the condition being treated (acute or chronic), back, front, torso, limbs or sense organs.

Resistance is Fortuitous

If there is resistance due to a node, push through the resistant part and come back to the required depth. When resistance is encountered, you may have to rotate the needle vigorously to break the nodule and resolve Stagnation in order to relieve the pain. Resistance due to adhesions or nodes can be so severe that the needle will bend. In this case the needle will require a stronger grip to push it through the blockage. Such strong resistance is fortuitous and it is often a 'eureka moment' as it is usually an indication that this is the point that will give the most effective therapeutic result and stop the pain. Tell your client that this is the point that will make all the difference and have them check what their pain reference score is at that moment. It should have decreased to at least 3-4 on a scale of 10. This is your 'internal cartwheel moment' so be sure to get the feedback as it will boost your confidence and improve future results too.

> **Tip:** By highlighting the process, and particularly by indicating the specific points that are taking the pain away, your client will be mesmerised and more likely to tell other potential clients about this miraculous form of acupuncture.

Needle resistance at a very superficial level can sometimes occur as a result of the skin at the insertion site becoming hard and tight due to the shock of the needle. In this case, the needle should be removed and reinserted. It will be obvious the way that the skin remains tight around the needle and lifts with it that this is a case of shock and tension in the epidermis rather than specifically indicating an Ahshi point. Rub around the point and reinsert the needle in a slightly different place. It should now pass through much easier.

Feel for a 'small fish' as described above. This is why abdominal acupuncture needling requires a very gentle sliding motion down the handle of the needle so that you can tune into the slightest anomalies as it passes through the relevant depths.

Check with your client with regards to how their pain is now. On a reference scale of 1-10 how has the pain changed? As you make more subtle adjustments keep checking with the client until the pain level has markedly improved. If there is no dramatic change and the needle appears to be at the right location and depth then leave it. If the pain moves then follow it, i.e. add more needles in the areas the pain has moved to until it is gone (see chapter 9, *Putting it all Together*, for more details!)

If pain moves from the shoulder to the lateral aspect of the upper arm along the Yangming meridian around LI 14 (Binao), then insert a needle approximately 0.2 cun distal to the shoulder point St 24 (Huaroumen) on a line between it and the elbow point Ab 1. If the pain then moves to the elbow, needle the relevant point around the elbow point (Ab 1) as there should be an Ahshi point there. Keep checking with your client, where the pain is after each additional needle. If the pain moves again, then chase it until it has gone!

> **Tip:** Remain calm and attentive to your client if the pain is moving as you perform AA, Communicate at each stage as you follow the pain. This will benefit your future treatments and it will emphasise to you and your client the subtle power of AA.

Adjust the needles as required. Add more needles to the relevant areas to treat Ahshi points and stop the pain. Feel for the arrival of De-Qi in the form of a small amount of resistance or tugging. The client does not necessarily need to experience Qi. Some clients with a better awareness of their body will feel the movement of Qi in the form of warmth and tingling or of rushes in the area of the body that is being mirrored by the turtle hologram.

Adjusting the Needle Depth

When withdrawing the needle to a shallower depth, it is important to do so in a controlled manner so as not to completely pull the needle out. Use your middle finger to push gently on the skin as your forefinger and thumb hold the handle and gently pull the needle up to the desired depth (see fig 6.3). You may have to fine tune the needle depth at Ahshi points a number of times before getting the desired result. During this stage of the treatment, it is vital that you maintain your focus and send your intention into the needle. It doesn't matter if the needles look haphazard as long as the pain is reduced, changed or ameliorated.

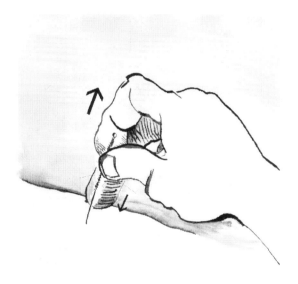

Fig 6.3. Controlled needle withdrawal to new depth method

Also, remember that, unlike traditional acupuncture, AA's results and therapeutic effect can change dramatically with minute alterations in depth and or location of the needles. So stay focused, be patient and get feedback when you are fine tuning (particularly Ahshi) points.

By following the above process you should find the right depth for the desired effect. At the beginning, don't worry too much that you might miss the subtle hints as to what is correct. Use each patient to enhance your experience and be aware of the correct depth that you will expect to need to go to to fix the pain. With the passing of time and many successful treatments, you will recognise these indicators from the feedback of the needle.

Aspects to Remember:

- Needles should be retained for 20-40 mins depending on whether the treatment is a reducing or tonifying one;
- If your client is not in pain at the time of treatment, then trust your intuition. Use all the steps above to localise the area in which the pain usually occurs. If all the indicators are telling you that this is the right place to treat for their problem, then be confident that the pain won't return as quickly as previously and that the intensity or the area affected by the pain will be reduced and/or changed;
- Occasionally results are not obvious for 24-48 hours. You may have to add needles around Ahshi points to be certain of getting the best result possible;
- Don't thrust or twirl needles to stimulate except when there is an adhesion that is resisting the needle. This is often the case where

there is an Ahshi point and by breaking up the adhesion the pain will disappear;

- A heat lamp is always nice for the client (except where there is Excessive Yang).

Concluding the Treatment

Once the needles are all in place and you are happy that the client has got the best results, leave your patient in a warm, comfortable room for between 20-40 minutes. The usual treatment time is about 30 minutes.

Once this time is completed, remove the needles from top to bottom and from outside to inside. If any of the points bleed, simply close them with cotton wool. If there is a haematoma apply some arnica cream and advise the client that they will most likely get a bruise that will be colourful rather than painful.

Bruises at Ren 12 (Zhongwan) may cause some minor headaches or palpitations and the area should not be needled again until the bruise has disappeared. A bruise at Ren 4 may cause some urinary disturbance and should not be needled again until it is completely gone. Bruises elsewhere seldom cause any adverse effects. Advise your client to apply arnica cream to the bruise a couple of times a day to speed up the recovery.

Remind your client that they might feel very tired after their treatment and to have a good night's sleep. As with other forms of acupuncture, abdominal can aggravate a condition in the short term though this is less likely to happen with AA in most cases.

Pain levels and mobility should improve over the next 24-48 hours. It is advisable to see clients in severe pain or with chronic conditions of a long duration twice a week for the first 3-4 weeks.

Summary of Topics Covered in this Chapter

We covered all aspects of how you should conduct an AA treatment including:

- The needle sequence for AA
- Managing your client in order to get the best feedback regarding their changes in pain
- How to recognise and needle Ahshi points in a way that will give the best therapeutic results possible
- How to manipulate AA needles to find the correct depth for your client's condition
- The subtleties of AA needle sensation from the perspective of the client and more importantly the therapist.

Chapter 7: Prescriptions: What's the Point?

Learning Objectives

This chapter is geared towards showing you a number of generalised or empirical prescriptions used for treating some painful conditions such as Bi Syndrome. They are the prerequisites for treating all kinds of painful conditions, which will be covered in chapter 8, *Abdominal Acupuncture Prescriptions for Frequently Seen Painful Conditions*.

Many of these empirical prescriptions were developed by Professor Bo to treat pain and move Qi and Blood thus facilitating subsequent needles to address specific painful conditions. You will also learn prescriptions that are nourishing for the whole body and those which treat particular aspects of Qi, Blood, Essence and Zang Fu organ health, therefore restoring harmony and balance to the body.

General Considerations

These prescriptions will help to give an understanding of how and why prescriptions in the aforementioned chapter 8 are formulated the way that they are. They will also enable you to develop a further appreciation of the power of AA and its effectiveness in treating a wide variety of ailments. It should also be apparent after reading chapter 4, *Points of the Abdomen,* how AA utilises these powerful points to give wide-ranging and dynamic results.

(Note: Prescription functions have been sourced from a number of places - Dr. Han Yan, personal communication; Lore, R. (2005); Ryan, P. M.S. L.AC. (2009); Yang. C 2012.)

Abdominal Acupuncture Prescriptions

Bringing Qi Home (also known as 'Guiding Qi to the Source')

Ren 12 (Zhongwan), Ren 10 (Xiawan), Ren 6 (Qihai) and Ren 4 (Guanyuan) (see Fig 7.1).

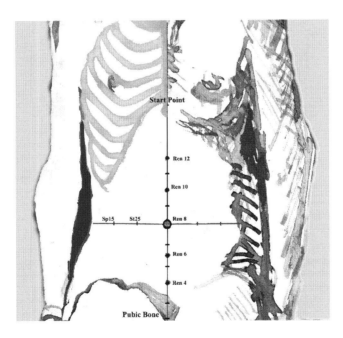

Fig 7.1. Bringing Qi Home /Guiding Qi to the Source

Function

This combination serves to promote the postnatal Qi (from the Spleen) to strengthen and benefit the pre-heaven Qi (Yuan) and thus send it home to the source, i.e. the Kidneys. It nourishes Bone, muscle and tendons. These points can treat diseases of the Heart and Lung, regulate the Spleen and Stomach and tonify the Liver and Kidneys.

Explanation

Ren 12 (Zhongwan) is the front Mu point of the Stomach. Ren 10 (Xiawan) also affects the Stomach and Spleen function as the 'sea of water & grain' thus nourishing postnatal Qi. They regulate the middle Jiao and assist the Lung in its function of dispersing and descending Qi.

Ren 6 (Qihai) is the 'Sea of Qi'. It fosters the original Qi as well as nourishing the Spleen and it tonifies the Qi and Yang of the Kidneys. Ren 4 (Guanyuan) is the 'Gate of the Original Qi' and invigorates the Kidney and Lung while benefiting the Spleen. It supplements the original Qi, Essence and tonifies Yang.

Thus, Ren 6 (Qihai) and Ren 4 (Guanyuan) help to consolidate the pre-heaven Qi of the Kidneys. They supplement Qi, Blood, Jing, Essence and ultimately Yin and Yang of the Kidneys and the entire body.

Needle Depths

Middle level 0.5-1.0 cun.

Comments

This is a frequently used prescription. It moves Qi throughout the abdomen and is an invigorating and nourishing treatment. I use this prescription in 85-90% of my treatments.

Heaven & Earth / Sky-Ground

Ren 12 (Zhongwan) & Ren 4 (Guanyuan) (see Fig 7.2).

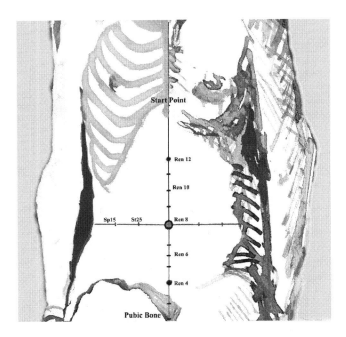

Fig 7.2. Heaven & Earth / Sky-Ground

Function

Invigorate the Spleen and tonify the Kidney.

Explanation

Ren 12 (Zhongwan) is the front Mu point of the Stomach. The Stomach and Spleen function is to 'transform and transport' essential nutrients and, therefore, nourish post-heaven Qi.

Ren 4 (Guanyuan) is the front Mu point of the Small Intestine. This is where the original Qi accumulates, so it invigorates the Kidney and thus pre-heaven Qi.

Both these points strengthen the Kidneys, tonify Qi and save the Yang.

Needle Depths

Middle level 0.5-1.0cun

Comments

This prescription can be used where there is not such a strong need for strengthening the Spleen and Kidneys. It can be used to nourish the Kidneys and to balance (fire) Heart and (water) Kidney energy. This is useful where the client is a little deficient and needs tonification. The combination is particularly beneficial where there is an element of anxiety and fear as these points have a strong calming effect. In these cases clients usually prefer fewer needles.

CASE STUDY: Cocaine Anxiety

I remember a client I had some years ago. He was a young man in his 20's who had been abusing cocaine and methadone (a prescription opioid medication often used in drug clinics as part of drug detoxification) for a number of years. He was extremely edgy, irritable and was suffering from severe anxiety and bouts of debilitating paranoia.

He was not very excited about the prospect of having acupuncture, and when I suggested I was going to use AA he expressed his lack of enthusiasm in no uncertain terms. I agreed that I would only use two points, and I indicated to him what he might feel by quickly pushing my index finger into his Stomach about 1cm and pulling it back just as quickly.

He was happy enough to give it a try. I used the 'Heaven and Earth' prescription (see Fig 7.2) and within minutes he was calm and he drifted off. After the 30 minute session he said he felt much more relaxed as if he was 'stoned'. He was delighted I had persuaded him to try acupuncture and his anxiety and paranoia improved to a very tolerable level within a few more weeks of treatment.

Abdominal Four Gates

Bilateral St 24 (Huaroumen) and St 26 (Wailing) (see Fig 7.3).

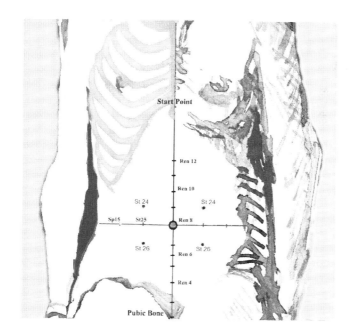

Fig 7.3. Abdominal Four Gates

Function

This prescription regulates the circulation of Qi and Blood to drain the channels and collaterals. It makes Qi and Blood rich and distributes meridian Qi to the upper and lower distal ends of the limbs. It also moves Zang Fu organ Qi smoothly throughout the body. These four points can treat all areas of the body. This combination can also be used to reduce high Blood pressure.

Explanation

St 24 (Huaroumen) regulates Qi and directs it through the upper limbs;

St 26 (Wailing) regulates Qi and directs it through the lower limbs.

Needle Depths

To act on the regulatory system, these points need to be needled to a depth of 0.5-1.0cun.

Comments

The abdominal four gates also has a great emotional impact and can be used to treat anxiety, stress, mania and depression. This prescription is often used at the initial stages (first six months) of treating those recovering from sequella due to Wind stroke.

Regulating Spleen Qi

Bilateral Sp 15 (Daheng) (see Fig 7.4).

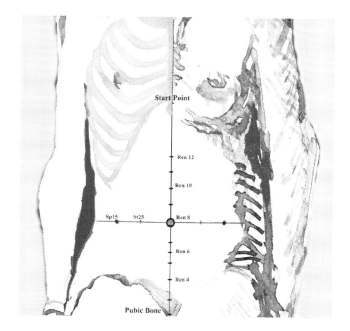

Fig 7.4. Regulating Spleen Qi

Function

Regulates the Spleen to invigorate its function of eliminating Dampness, nourishing the muscles and lubricating the joints.

Explanation

Sp 15 (Daheng) is located on the ascending and descending portions of the colon. Therefore it regulates the middle Jiao, invigorates Spleen function and assists with clearing Dampness while nourishing the muscles and limbs and lubricating the joints.

Comments

Sp 15 (Daheng) is often used to relieve spasm in the back and to treat back pain and reduce swelling. It also has a strong impact on emotional disharmonies such as sadness and sighing.

Harmonising the Middle Jiao

St 25 (Tianshu) and Sp 15 (Daheng) (See Fig 7.5).

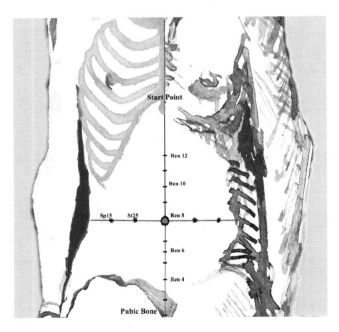

Fig 7.5. Harmonising the middle Jiao

Function

These 4 points harmonise the middle Jiao and regulate digestion.

Explanation

As the front Mu point of the Large Intestine, St 25 (Tianshu) it is capable of regulating the 3 Jiao's - upper Jiao via Lungs, middle Jiao through the Stomach, its associated organ, and the lower Jiao by virtue of its anatomical location and function. It has the function of clearing Heat through the Large Intestine. (Lore. R. 2005)

Sp 15 (Daheng) also has a regulatory function over the middle Jiao and the intestines and it clears Dampness and nourishes the Spleen.

Comments

Harmonising the middle Jiao can be used for all kinds of digestive problems and is often used in conjunction with 'Bringing Qi Home' to treat obesity and to help with weight management.

General Tonification and Immune System Boosting Prescription

Points used are 'Bringing Qi Home', Ren 12 (Zhongwan), Ren 10 (Xiawan), Ren 6 (Qihai) and Ren 4 (Guanyuan), combined with St 24 (Huaroumen) and St 26 (Wailing), see Fig 7.6.

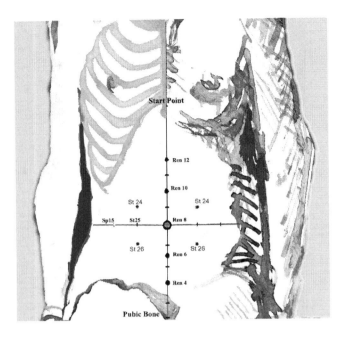

Fig 7.6. General tonification and immune system boosting prescription

Function

This combination of 'Bringing Qi Home' and the four gates nourishes the Spleen and Kidneys by sending the postnatal Qi to invigorate the prenatal Qi. It opens the middle Jiao and descends the Lung Qi. This prescription also dredges the meridians and invigorates Qi and Blood and benefits the emotions. These 8 points give a strong boost to the immune system.

Explanation

See above explanations for 'Bringing Qi Home' and the abdominal four gates.

Comments

'Bringing Qi Home' puts nutrient Qi into the Kidneys, thus improves Essence and keeps the body healthy.

The four gates can maintain a healthy blood pressure and is a powerful treatment for emotional issues including mania and depression, which if untreated can lead to a myriad of physical manifestations.

Rheumatism/Arthritis Prescription

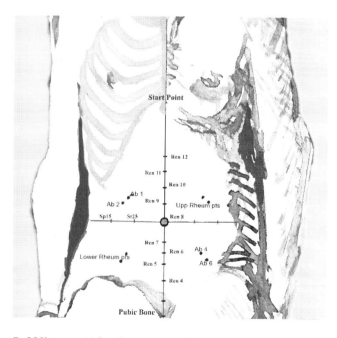

Fig 7.7 Rheumatism / Arthritis Prescription 'Feng Shi Dian'

These points are collectively known as Feng Shi Dian. They are bilateral, upper rheumatism Ab 1 (elbow) points and upper lateral rheumatism Ab 2 (wrist) points, lower rheumatism Ab 4 (knee) and lower lateral rheumatism Ab 6 (ankle) points (see Fig 7.7).

Function

Together these points function to dredge the meridians and collaterals, and clear Wind and Dampness from the joints, thus eliminating swelling and alleviating pain.

Explanation

A look at the Ba Gua hologram shows that left side elbow Ab1 point (Shang Fen Xi) is in the Gua of Kun, which dominates over the Stomach and Spleen. For this reason, this point also treats Spleen Qi problems and thus regulates and clears Dampness. Dui dominates lower Jiao. Ab 1 (Shang Fen Xi), also known as elbow point (Ab 1) on the right, dominates over the middle Jiao as it's in the Gua is Xun which encapsulated the Liver and thus has Wind clearing properties. Ab 4 knee point (Xia Fen Shi) on the right is in the Gua of Gen, which dominates over the upper Jiao. Ab 4 on the left is in the Gua of Qian, which houses the Large Intestine and Lung which both have eliminatory functions of fluids and thus Dampness.

Comments

These points should be needled to a depth of 1.0-1.5 cun to work on the Zang Fu organs at the Ba Gua (earth) level.

Bi Syndrome Pain in the Upper and or Lower Parts of the Body

Abdominal four gates bilateral St 24 (Huaroumen) and St 26 (Wailing) combined with the rheumatism points bilateral, upper rheumatism (elbow) Ab 1 points and upper lateral rheumatism (wrist) Ab 2 points (see Fig 7.8).

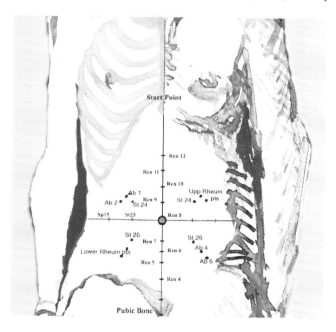

Fig. 7.8. Abdominal 4 gates with Feng Shi Dian points

This combination of points treats all over arthritic type Bi Syndrome and/or if the pain is of a wandering Bi type nature.

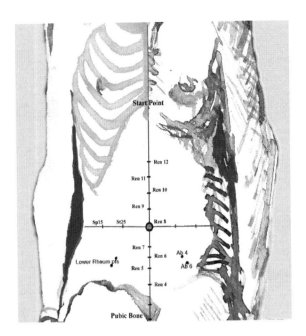

Fig 7.9. Lower Rheumatism / Arthritis Prescription

If the pain is only affecting the lower joints, just use lower rheumatism points, i.e. Ab 4 (knee) and Ab 6 (ankle) bilaterally as in Fig 7.9 above.

If the pain is only affecting the upper area, just use upper rheumatism points, i.e. Ab 1 (elbow) and Ab 2 (wrist) as in Fig 7.10 below.

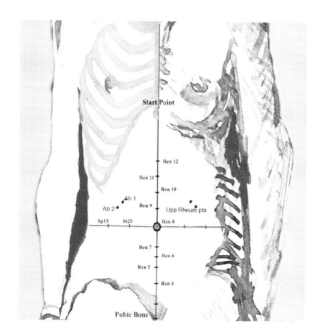

Fig 7.10. Upper Rheumatism / Arthritis Prescription

If the condition is acute with swelling and inflammation, then include Sp 15 (Daheng) bilaterally.

Diamond Treatment

Ren 12 (Zhongwan), Ren 4 (Guanyuan) Fig 7.11.1, or Ren 6 (Qihai) (Fig 7.11.2) and St 25 (Tianshu) bilaterally.

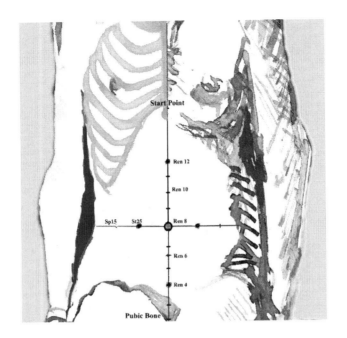

Fig 7.11.1. Diamond treatment with Ren 4 (Guanyuan)

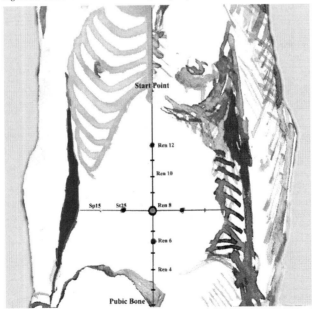

Fig 7.11.2. Diamond treatment with Ren 6 (Qihai)

Function

These points promote the circulation of Qi and Blood in the abdomen, invigorate the Spleen and Kidney and enhance the effect of subsequent needles used.

Comment

This is a frequently used prescription. St 25 (Tianshu) makes the connection between East and West. It is also capable of regulating the 3 Burners while Ren 12 (Zhongwan) and Ren 4 (Guanyuan) or Ren 6 (Qihai) connects south and north, Yang and Yin aspects.

Different Needle Formats

Needles can be added in any of the various formats (see below) to enhance the effect of the treatment. The main point should be needled first, and subsequent or secondary needles can be added diagonally or in a line. These can be changed but the main point should remain the central point.

Triangular Method

Needles can be placed in a triangular format 0.1-0.5 cun apart (depending on how far the pain radiates from the source) with the main point being at the apex of the triangle. This format is often used on Ahshi points such as when treating knee, shoulder or, as in the case below, elbow pain (see Fig 7.12.1).

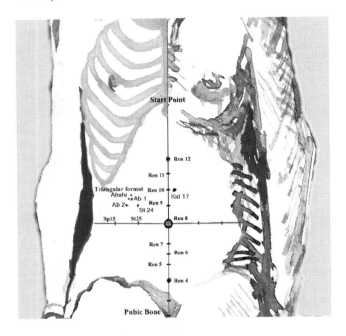

Fig 7.12.1. Triangular needle format at Ab 1 elbow point

Three Star Needle Method

This method uses the centre needle as the main acupuncture point with a needle at either side in a straight line 0.3-0.5cun apart. This format is used to reinforce Ahshi points, particularly where the condition is moving in a line, such as with sciatic pain moving along the UB meridian from UB 36 (Chengfu) to UB 40 (Weizhong) (see Fig 7.12.2). This format is often used to chase the pain away as it moves with the progression of an AA treatment (see Chapter 6, *Abdominal Acupuncture Treatment Protocols*).

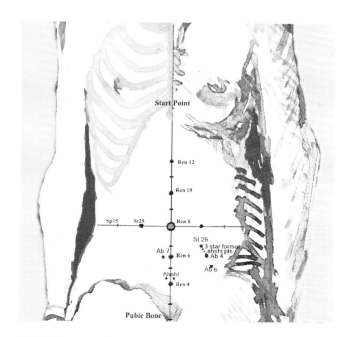

Start Point

Ren 12

Ren 10

Sp15   St25   Ren 8

St 26
3 star format
Ab 7   ahshi pts
Ren 6   Ab 4
Ab 6
Ahshi
Ren 4

Pubic Bone

Fig 7.12.2. 3star format from UB 36 (Chengfu) to UB 40 (Weizhong)

Plum Blossom Method

Here four needles surround the main needle in the centre to reinforce the treatment (see Fig 7.12.3).

The number of needles used to reinforce or improve the effect on Ahshi points can be more than the above stated. Other shapes, such as the Y shape that is a triangle plus one needle, can also be produced. The diamond method sees an extra needle at the opposite end to the apex of the triangle.

All of the above methods are intended to improve the result of the treatment and relieve pain in a particular area of the body, especially if the pain is radiating across a large area such as the knee, hip, shoulder, etc.

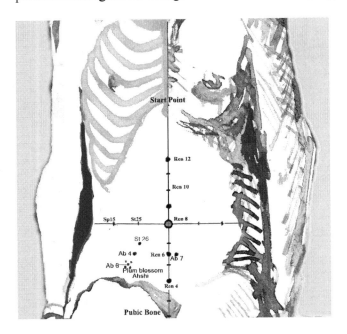

Fig 7.12.3. Plum blossom format around the ankle point (Ab 6)

Reducing Excess

When clearing Excess, needle shallow with thicker gauge needles and use more needles for a shorter period.

Tonifying Deficiency

To tonify use smaller gauge needles. Use fewer needles and needle deeper for a longer duration of time.

Summary of Topics Covered in this Chapter

- The structure and function of nine generalised prescriptions
- Why these prescriptions function the way they do
- When these prescriptions might be used
- Different supplementary needle formats and when they are used
- Tonification and reducing methods with AA.

Chapter 8: Abdominal Acupuncture Prescriptions for Frequently Seen Painful Conditions

Learning Objectives

In this chapter I offer a number of suggestions for treating frequently seen painful conditions. I will then give real case histories of treating these problems to support and emphasise the different potential approaches available to you when treating each of the conditions. This chapter is relatively longer than preceding chapters due to the comprehensive nature of the case studies included, which are contained in each of the sub-sections. However, now that you've arrived at the latter part of this book, you should be able to confidently treat most painful conditions described here. After leading you by the hand in formulating prescriptions for a range of frequently seen problems I will loosen the apron strings, so to speak, so that you can produce your own methods of treating the remaining problems highlighted here.

General Considerations

All of the prescriptions follow on from those presented in the previous chapter, *What's the Point?* They have been refined through my own practice and Centreforce training courses over the years to give the best results and can be used in combination with traditional acupuncture or independently. These prescriptions have proven to give consistent and reliable results over the years that I have been practising and teaching abdominal acupuncture.

The needle depths should serve as a guide. However, they will vary with subjects of different weight and depending on the severity and duration of their conditions. The main thing to be aware of when trying to decide what depth is correct is the feedback that you get from your patients. If their pain has improved, then you are at the right depth. You should also let the needle guide you as described in chapter 6, *Abdominal Acupuncture Treatment Protocols*. When you first feel some resistance and you know the needle is within the level you are treating, then trust that you are at the correct depth. As your intuition develops, this will become second nature.

I have divided this chapter into subsections to allow you to work through each condition presented and in this format it allows you to dip in and out of relevant sub-sections as you require.

General Considerations to help you Formulate Prescriptions

- When there is Qi Stagnation involved use Ren 6 (Qihai) to invigorate and move Qi;
- If there is Blood stasis present use Ren 4 (Guanyuan) to nourish and move Blood;
- Where there is Dampness affecting the whole body use **Feng Shi Dian** bilaterally
- Upper rheumatism Ab 1 (elbow) points and upper lateral rheumatism Ab 2 (wrist) points. Lower rheumatism Ab 4(knee) and lower lateral rheumatism Ab 6 (ankle) points;

- If there is Dampness in the upper body only (i.e. above the waist) use bilateral, upper rheumatism (elbow) points, i.e. Ab 1 and upper lateral rheumatism (wrist) points Ab 2;
- For Dampness below the waist **lower Feng Shi Dian** points, Ab 4 (lower rheumatism point) and Ab 6 (lower lateral rheumatism points) bilaterally;
- When a condition is acute, and there is inflammation, Ren 9 (Shuifen) should be used to resolve swelling;
- Sp 15 (Daheng) should be used for chronic problems where there is a weakness of the muscles and joints.

A Note on Suggested Prescriptions used for Frequently Seen Conditions

Each of the suggested prescriptions below will start with a comprehensive treatment that should have a good therapeutic result. The initial treatments have served me well and are always reliable. I also provide more minimal treatments for each of the conditions. These will be successful most of the time and will often give the same powerful initial results but may not have the same longevity as the more comprehensive prescriptions. On occasions, I will offer a third option using only Ahshi points. These prescriptions will also often work and can give the same results but generally these options are best used where there are no other underlying root causes for the pain.

I want to provide you with a number of options to allow you to explore different methods and approaches so that abdominal acupuncture can also be used in a more time efficient manner. The various options also highlight some of the different approaches that can be taken and indicate the fluid nature of abdominal acupuncture. These prescriptions are by no means the only options available for each condition listed, but they are the most likely to provide the best efficacy in the majority of cases.

The more minimal treatments are ideal for such settings as communal acupuncture clinics where time is of the essence. They are also suited to those with a serious fear of needles or for those with a weak constitution.

******Section One ******

Abdominal Acupuncture Prescriptions for Upper Back / Neck Problems

Option 1

- Bringing Qi Home, Ren 12 (Zhongwan), Ren10 (Xiawan), Ren6 (Qihai) and Ren4 (Guanyuan);
- Kid 13 (Qixue) bilaterally;
- This will supplement the Spleen and Kidney to nourish muscle, Bone and thus the vertebra in the upper back and neck. Kid 13 (Qixue) will assist in the function of nourishing Marrow and, therefore, will indirectly benefit the neck and upper back;
- St 24 (Huaroumen) should be used bilaterally if the problem is affecting both sides of the upper back or unilaterally if one-sided on the affected side;

- When treating pain around GB 21 (Jianjing), Ahshi points will most likely be found in the region of the shoulder St 24 (Huaroumen), possibly 0.2-0.3 cun medially to this point;
- Ahshi points in the vicinity of Kid 17 (Shangqu) can also treat pain in the region of GB21 (Jianjing);
- When the pain is located along the upper back, covering a large area incorporating points such as UB11 (Dazhu), SI 15 (Jianzhongshu), SI 14 (Jianweishu), use Kid 17 (Shangqu) and local Ahshi points;
- If the pain is located along the Huato Jiaji line rather than the UB channel use Ahshi points between the Kidney and Ren channels;
- For pain along the neck between cervical vertebrae 1 (C-1) and C-7 use relevant Ahshi points between Ren 11 (Jianli) and Ren 10 (Xiawan). If the discomfort is located at GB 20 (Fengchi) this will most likely be best addressed using an Ahshi point around Kid 18 (Shiguan);
- In the case of acute conditions, use Ren 9 (Shuifen) which should be needled deep to activate the Zang Fu function of clearing inflammation;
- If the discomfort covers a larger area such as between GB 20 (Fengchi) and GB 21 (Jianjing) then a number of needles may be needed around St 24 (Huaroumen), Kid 17 (Shangqu) and/or Kid 18 (Shiguan) (see Fig 8.1).

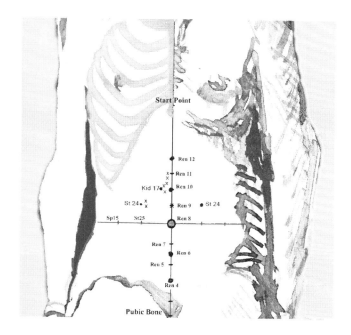

Fig 8.1. AA Prescriptions Option 1: for upper back / neck problems (Note X indicates possible Ahshi locations.)

Option 2

Abdominal Acupuncture Prescription for Upper Back / Neck Pain - A Little Bit of Minimalism:

If the patient has strong constitutional Qi and/or is young with no deep rooted cause for the problem and if there are no other symptoms you can just use points above the umbilicus, i.e.:

- Ren 12 (Zhongwan), Ren 10 (Xiawan);
- St 24 (Huaroumen) bilaterally or unilaterally if the pain is one-sided, on the affected side;
- Kid 17 (Shangqu) will address problems in upper back and the base of the neck (as described above in option 1);

- Locate and treat Ahshi points in and around St 24 (Huaroumen), Ren 10 (Xiawan) and Kid 17 (Shangqu). Use whatever format to address the Ahshi points, area and size. For example, it may be necessary to put a triangular or **Y** type format in the vicinity of Kid 17 (Shangqu);
- Adjust the needle depths and fine tune as above for best results or until the pain has gone (see Fig 8.2).

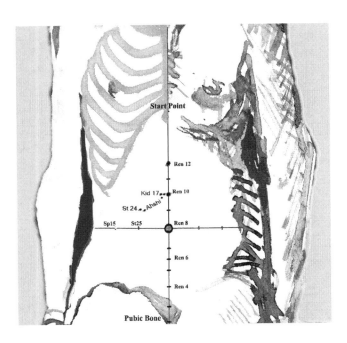

Fig 8.2 Option 2: for right sided upper back / neck problems

Option 3

Abdominal Acupuncture Prescriptions for Upper Back / Neck Pain - A Little Bit more Minimalism:

- Isolate and treat Ahshi points in and around St 24 (Huaroumen), Ren 10 (Xiawan) and Kid 17 (Shangqu). Use whatever needle format that best address the Ahshi points, area and pain;
- Adjust the needle depths and fine tune as above for best results.

CASE STUDY: A Busy Chef's Neck and Shoulder Pain

Sally first consulted me through a chance meeting. We were both guests at a dinner party and when I told her what I did she revealed that she was currently attending a physiotherapist for severe neck and shoulder pain that radiated down her right arm. The pain was bad enough to warrant using the most powerful over-the-counter painkillers and anti-inflammatories. The condition was impacting on both Sally's social and professional life. Physiotherapy and dry needling (trigger point) would give short-term relief of 2-3 days. However, if Sally had a busy work schedule, this relief was only hours rather than days.

I agreed to treat her with abdominal acupuncture. On her first visit she also had a bad bout of sinusitis and was feeling very congested from the forehead to below the eyes. Sally was in a lot of pain especially from GB 20 (Fengxi) to GB 21, SI 13 (Quyuan) and on a line through SI 11 (Tianzong) and SI 12 (Bingfeng). She also had an Ahshi point around UB 43 (Gaohangshu). The whole area was tight and always felt tense even when there was no major pain. The treatment principle was to move Qi and Blood to nourish the muscles in the area affected. It was also important to clear the sinuses that had become troublesome in recent months.

Palpation revealed a number of nodules between Ren 10 (Xiawan) and Ren 11 (Jianli) along both the Conception Vessel and the Kidney meridian. There were no anomalies felt around the shoulder point at St 24 (Huaroumen) or along the route of the elbow (Ab1) and wrist (Ab 2) points on the right-hand side. Between Ren10 (Xiawan) and Ren 9 (Shuifen) lateral to the Kidney meridian on the right, there was one large solid nodule that represented the blockage at UB43 (Gaohangshu). There were some spongy superficial nodes just above Ren 12 (Zhongwan), suggesting Phlegm in the sinus area of the face.

The prescription used was 'Bringing Qi Home' with Ren 12 (Zhongwan), Ren 10 (Xiawan), Ren 6 (Qihai) and Ren 4 (Guanyuan) to move the postnatal Qi to the Kidney and supplement pre-heaven and Spleen Qi. Kid 17 (Shangqu) was used on the right side with two Ahshi needles in a triangular format to break up the nodes in the area. Spleen 15 (Daheng) was chosen to nourish the muscles and clear Damp. Kidney 13 (Qixue) was needled bilaterally to nourish Marrow and to help relieve the neck pain. The Ahshi point located between Ren 10 (Xiawan) and Ren 9 (Shuifen) along the Kidney meridian was punctured.

The needle met strong resistance at a depth of approximately 0.3-0.4 cun. The nodule needed a lot of strong needle stimulation to break it down, and the needle was left for 15 minutes before more stimulation was given to further reduce this stubborn nodule. A further two needles were added laterally and medially approximately 0.2 cun apart on a horizontal line, which addressed the scapular pain. This combination brought the pain here down from 10 to a very comfortable 3. Sally commented that she felt a lot of heat radiating from the point where the pain had been around the scapula.

As there were no abnormalities felt around St 24 (Huaroumen) this point was not used. Instead, because of the recent sinus problems, it was decided to use a point 0.2 cun medial and inferior to it, which is anatomically in line with Lu1 (Zhongfu). This point was needled to a depth of 0.4 cun to help move Lung Qi downwards and restore normal function to the sinuses. The Ahshi points felt laterally and superior to Ren 12 (Zhongwan) were needled more superficially to benefit directly the nasal passages (see Fig 8.3).

Four more treatments were done for Sally over the next three weeks. The sinus problem was treated twice. On two occasions the scapular pain was no longer present and Sally had some pain only in the shoulder. This was treated using St 24 (Huaroumen), the shoulder point, which relieved the pain. Sally occasionally has a treatment after a busy week. However, she has been pain-free for the most part, a result that she never expected after getting only minimal relief from two years of physiotherapy and dry needling.

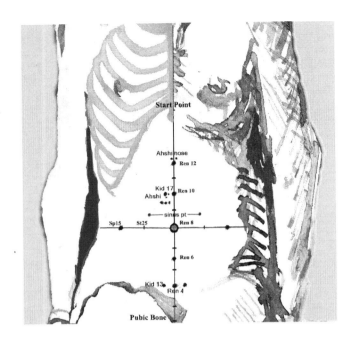

Fig 8.3. AA Prescription for 'A Busy Chef's Neck and Shoulder Pain'

CASE STUDY: Bob the Builder with a Bad Back

Bob, a bricklayer by trade, had chronic pain due to a slipped disc at thoracic vertebra no. 3 (T-3). He was prescribed Diaphene and was using *Nurofen Plus* and other strong codeine-based over-the-counter medication to try and control the pain. As a result of almost eighteen months using medication, he had Spleen Qi Vacuity and Kidney Yang Vacuity.

He was nervous and didn't want to have his back needled after a previous treatment with a physiotherapist had caused him to faint. He had tried chiropractic and osteopathic therapy and had not responded to either.

The treatment began with the prescription of 'Bringing Qi Home' with Ren 12 (Zhongwan), Ren 10 (Xiawan), Ren 6 (Qihai) and Ren 4 (Guanyuan) to strengthen the Kidney and Spleen Qi and nourish Kidney Yang. Kid 17 (Shangqu) was used bilaterally to enhance the effect of the needles at Ren 10 (Xiawan) of invigorating the Spleen and Stomach. Ahshi points were located between Ren 9 (Shuifen) and Ren 10 (Xiawan). These points were needled to a depth of 0.4 - 0.5 cun to work on the affected disc at T-3. Huato Jiaji points in the location of T-3 were also stimulated by needling points about 0.2cun lateral to the midline and the depth was again approximately 0.4 - 0.5 cun. St 25 (Tianshu) and St 24 (Huaroumen) were also needled bilaterally to ease pain and spasm of the large muscles (Latissimus Dorsi) of the back.

Within minutes of starting the treatment the pain moved and after some fine tuning of the needles the pain had totally gone. He returned for his second session four days later and was delighted that he had not had to use any medication and had been able to enjoy normal activities. Bob's digestion had also improved and he was not suffering from bouts of nausea. The treatment protocol remained the same for the first three treatments (see Fig 8.4).

Throughout the final four sessions the Kid 17 (Shangqu) points were removed as the medication that had weakened the Spleen and Stomach was no longer necessary after the first abdominal acupuncture session. St 25 (Tianshu) was also eliminated as it was doubling up in its action as the front Mu point of the Large Intestine. All other points remained the same although the number of Ahshi points was reduced from 3 to 1 (see fig 8.4).

Bob had a total of seven treatments and was able to return to work as a bricklayer.

Bob had another MRI scan following abdominal acupuncture treatment and the scan results testified that the disc had moved back into the correct position following a course of abdominal acupuncture. Eighteen months later Bob's back was still pain-free.

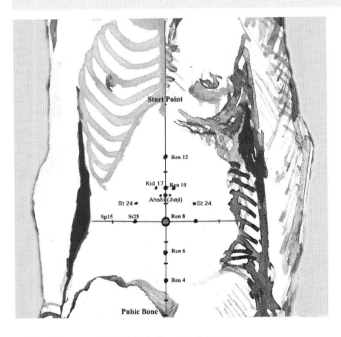

Fig 8.4. AA Prescription for 'Bob the Builder with a Bad Back'

******Section Two******

Abdominal Acupuncture Prescriptions to Treat Conditions of the Shoulders, Upper Limbs and Digits

In this section I will be addressing various conditions including:

- Frozen shoulder/shoulder pain;
- Shoulder and referred arm pain;
- Tennis elbow;
- Carpal tunnel syndrome/wrist pain;
- Arthritis or Bi Syndrome, and all kinds of problems affecting the hands, fingers and thumbs, including repetitive strain injury (RSI).

I will offer suggested treatments for each and then a minimal treatment as I have done above.

Shoulder Problems

Shoulder problems are commonly encountered in the clinic and, as the shoulders cover a relatively large area, treatments can vary with Ahshi points being found around the shoulder point, i.e. St 24 (Huaroumen), or in the vicinity of Kid 17 (Shangqu). Shoulder pain can often cause referred pain down the arm or into both the neck and head. If this is the case, then a more comprehensive treatment will be required until the pain becomes more localised. When the condition is new or acute and more localised, fewer needles will give good results unless there are complications.

Frozen Shoulder

This is a particularly painful condition and it can result in limited mobility, stiffness and referred pain. Often there will be a distinct temperature decrease felt on the abdomen around the shoulder point, i.e. St 24 (Huaroumen) on the affected side.

A Comprehensive Treatment for Frozen / Painful Shoulder

If the pain is chronic, and the client is Deficient, then it is worthwhile using the 'Bringing Qi Home / to the Source' prescription. If there is a temperature difference (i.e. Cold) around the shoulder area of the abdomen (St 24 Huaroumen), then there will be an element of external Cold invasion or Deficiency of Yang leading to internal Cold. In either case, heat should be applied to the relevant shoulder.

Prescription for Chronic Shoulder Pain:

- 'Bringing Qi Home / to the Source' i.e. Ren 12 (Zhongwan), Ren 10 (Xiawan), Ren 6 (Qihai) and Ren 4 (Guanyuan);
- Kid 17 (Shangqu) on the affected side;
- St 24 (Huaroumen) on the affected side. When the pain is covering a large area of the anterior and posterior of the shoulder a number of needles at various depths may be necessary in the area of St 24 (Huaroumen) to achieve a good result. See the case study in section one, above 'A Busy Chef's Upper Back and Shoulder Pain' and below 'A Case of Frozen Shoulder'.

CASE STUDY: A Case of Frozen Shoulder

Fred came for acupuncture as a result of his shoulder, which was progressively becoming more painful and less mobile by the day. He had gradually developed this problem and was having difficulty lifting his arm to the front or back. His main pain was on the Large Intestine (Hand Yangming) and Sanjiao (Hand Shao Yang) meridians. Heat packs gave some relief to this 34-year-old. He had a warm abdomen, in general, but the area around his right shoulder (St 24 Huaroumen) was palpably colder.

There was also an obvious nodule the size of a small pea. As Fred was otherwise very healthy a very minimal treatment was used - namely, Ren 12 (Zhongwan) and Ren 4 (Guanyuan) to connect the north and south. St 24 (Huaroumen) on the right was needled through the nodule to a depth of 0.4 cun and after it had dissipated the needle was withdrawn a little and left at a superficial depth of 0.2 cun.

On questioning Fred and getting him to rotate his arm he acknowledged that the pain at the front was almost totally gone. However, there was still some pain at the back of his shoulder. Another needle was inserted approximately 2 fen (0.2 cun) superior and lateral to St 24 (Huaroumen). This needle was left slightly deeper (due to the fact the pain was at the back of the shoulder) to give the best effect at approximately 0.3 cun (see Fig 8.5). When rotating his arm on this occasion, Fred reported minimal discomfort and he was left for 25 minutes with the needles in situ. A heat lamp was placed above the abdomen to warm the shoulder area and the point Ren 8 (Shenque), thus invigorating his body's Yang energy.

This treatment was repeated three more times and the shoulder problem was resolved completely.

Moxa can be used on the needles but as they were so superficial it was not practical. It was not necessary to use moxa on Ren 8 (Shenque) as the Yang Deficiency was only affecting the local area of the shoulder.

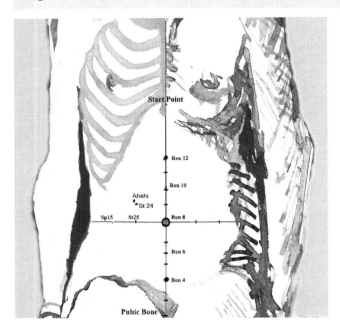

Fig 8.5. AA Prescription for 'A Case of Frozen Shoulder'

Prescription for Acute Shoulder Pain or Sports Injury:

- Ren 12 (Zhongwan);
- Ren 9 (Shuifen) at the acute stage, to relieve swelling and inflammation;
- Kid 17 (Shangqu) on the affected side;
- St 24 (Huaroumen) on the affected side;

~ 218 ~

- Locate the Ahshi points on the abdomen and adjust the depths or add needles in a format that best addresses the area of pain, e.g. a triangular format (see Fig 8.6).

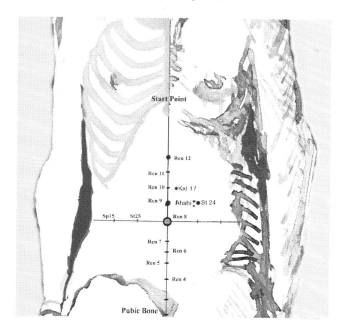

Fig 8.6. AA Prescription for treating acute shoulder pain

A More Minimal Prescription for Acute Shoulder Pain or Sports Injury:

- St 24 (Huaroumen) on the affected side;
- Locate the Ahshi points on the abdomen and adjust the depths or add needles in a format that best addresses the area of pain, e.g. a triangular format.

Prescription for Treating Shoulder and Referred Pain:

Shoulder and upper limb problems are treated similarly with more attention being focused on the relevant painful area.

- If the problem is of a chronic nature use 'Bringing Qi Home / to the Source', i.e. Ren 12 (Zhongwan), Ren 10 (Xiawan), Ren 6 (Qihai) and Ren 4 (Guanyuan);
- Kid 17 (Shangqu) on the affected side;
- When there is referred pain moving down the arm, it is essential to open the gate to move Qi from the Kidneys to the relevant shoulder and down the entire arm. This is achieved by needling the opposite or contra lateral Kid 17 (Shangqu) point;
- Then needle shoulder point, St 24 (Huaroumen);
- Ab 1 (elbow) and Ab 2 (wrist) points should be treated on the affected side when the whole arm is affected;
- If the pain only radiates as far as the intersection of the muscle deltoideus at the level of LI 14 (Binao), then only needle distally as far as Ab 1 elbow point;
- If the referred pain radiates past the elbow or changes and starts moving down the whole arm continue with needling wrist point Ab 2;
- When the pain is covering a large area of the anterior and posterior of the shoulder a number of needles at various depths may be necessary in the area of St 24 (Huaroumen) to achieve a good result. It may also be appropriate to use Kid 17 (Shangqu) on the affected side to completely remove the pain;
- Be mindful of the area you are treating. Locate the Ahshi points on the abdomen and adjust the depths or add needles to work at

multiple pain sites.(see case histories, 'A Case of Frozen Shoulder' and 'A Busy Chef's Upper Back and Shoulder Pain' above in section one of this chapter);

- Locate the Ahshi points in each of the relevant areas. Start with the shoulder and move distally towards the wrist or fingers. In this example, where pain is focused at the intersection of the muscle deltoideus at the level of LI 14 (Binao), locate the Ahshi approximately midway between shoulder point St 24 (Huaroumen) and Ab 1 elbow point;

- Treating the thumb will necessitate using the thumb point (Ab 3) while finger points will be found lateral to and between the level of the wrist (Ab 2) and the elbow point (Ab 1). These Ahshi points should only require very superficial needling to achieve the desired goal (see Fig 8.7).

It is possible to just needle the affected area of the body, such as the elbow point (Ab1) for elbow pain and get rid of the pain. From my experience, I find that it is best to move Qi through the whole area. This is more important for first treatments and particularly when you are familiarising yourself with abdominal acupuncture.

If the problem is due to Wind/Damp, then use rheumatism points (Feng Shi Dian). If there is a Bi Syndrome affecting only the upper part of the body (above the waist), just use Ab 1 and Ab 2 anti-arthritic points bilaterally (see fig 8.9) and include Ab 3 if the pain goes into the fingers. If the whole body is being affected then use all Feng Shi Dian points (see 'General Considerations' to help you formulate prescriptions above), or Damp only due to Spleen Deficiency use Sp 15 (Daheng).

Tip: When there are a number of Ahshi points detected and the pain is moving it is imperative that you maintain communication with your client. By checking with them how the pain has changed with each needle inserted and/or adjusted, you will get a comprehensive picture as to which needles are exerting the best results and where. You might have to come back to these needles later if the pain changes. If this happens, it will be very useful to know exactly what the effect is of each of the Ahshi needles.

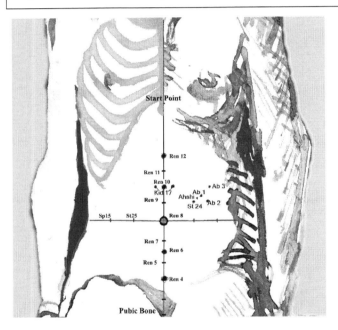

Fig 8.7. AA Prescription to treat shoulder and referred limb pain

Prescriptions to treat Tennis / Golfers Elbow and Other Types of Elbow Problems:

Tennis elbow can affect anywhere around the elbow, usually between the Large Intestine (hand Yangming) the Sanjiao (hand Shaoyang) or the

Small Intestine, 'SI' (hand Taiyang) meridians. This will be important both for the depth and the location of the needles around the elbow point Ab 1.

If you feel there is an element of Deficiency use the more comprehensive treatment as described below:

- 'Bringing Qi Home /to the Source', i.e. Ren 12 (Zhongwan), Ren 10 (Xiawan), Ren 6 (Qihai) and Ren 4 (Guanyuan);
- Kid 17 (Shangqu) contra–laterally;
- Then needle shoulder point St 24 (Huaroumen) Ab 1 (elbow) and Ab 2 (wrist) points on the affected side;
- Isolate the Ahshi points that best address the area of pain. They should be within a 0.5 cun radius of the Ab 1 (elbow) point, no matter where the elbow pain is originating. The depth will usually be less deep for the front Yangming area as opposed to the back SI (hand Taiyang) area of the elbow. See Fig 8.8, chapter 9, *Putting it all Together* and 'Ed's Elbow' below).

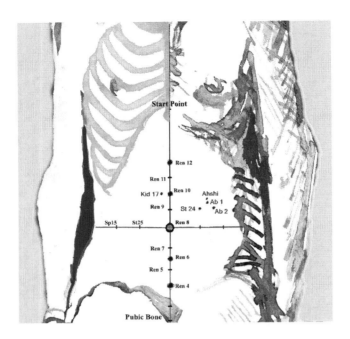

Fig 8.8. AA Prescription for treating elbow problems

CASE STUDY: Ed's Elbow

Ed, a 49-year-old graphic designer, had right elbow pain between the hand Yangming and Shaoyang meridians. The pain was sharp on occasion causing him to avoid certain movements, and the pain was particularly bad after a busy day using the computer mouse. There was a constant dull ache that was worse in wet weather, and he had to give up exercising at the gym as a result.

On his first visit he was in considerable pain and had no problem with putting a reference point score of 10 on his pain. Flexion with a lateral rotation caused pain that was easy to localise. Ren 12 (Zhongwan) and Ren 4 (Guanyuan) was chosen to strengthen the Spleen and Kidneys to nourish the joint and Bone. Kid 17 (Shangqu) was needled on the opposite side (left) to move Qi down the shoulder and through the entire right arm. The shoulder point St 24 (Huaroumen), elbow (Ab 1) and wrist (Ab 2) were all needled to the heaven level. The elbow point (Ab 1) was needled with a triangular formation with the Ahshi point at the apex. The Ahshi point had quite an obvious superficial nodule, as expected, just superior to the elbow point (Ab 1). This point was needled through the nodule that had put up quite a bit of resistance. The needling technique used was more aggressive than normal due to the nature of the resistance experienced at this point. The main Ahshi point was needled to a depth of 0.3-0.4 cun until it had passed through and broken down the nodule (by lifting thrusting and twirling the needle).

Immediately after, Ed was told to move his elbow in the same manner as he had done earlier. He experienced no pain and the needle was left at a superficial depth of 0.2 cun.

As this problem was due to Damp Bi Syndrome, Ab 1 (elbow) and Ab 2 (wrist) were included on the left side to a depth of 0.5 cun to clear the Dampness and nourish the joints (see Fig 8.9). Ed had three more treatments. The triangular needling at the elbow point was not necessary, and only Ab 1 was used on these occasions. Otherwise, the treatment remained the same. Ed has not had any elbow pain since. It has been two years since his first treatment.

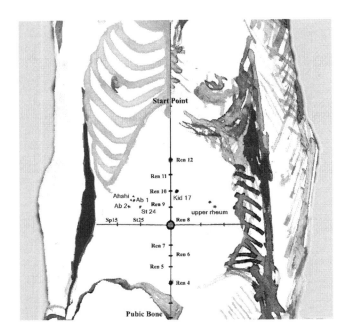

Fig 8.9. AA Prescription for 'Ed's Elbow Pain'

When there is Dampness involved such as with arthritis or other Bi Syndrome type conditions, use **Feng Shi Dian** points above the umbilicus.

- Bilateral, upper rheumatism (elbow) points, i.e. Ab 1 and upper lateral rheumatism (wrist) points Ab 2.

If this problem has no other causative factors such as Dampness, then a simple treatment as described below will give good results.

- Ren 12 (Zhongwan);
- St 24 (Huaroumen) and Ab 1 elbow point on the affected side;
- Isolate and treat the Ahshi points in the locality of Ab 1, using triangular or other formats as appropriate.

~ 226 ~

Carpal Tunnel Syndrome / Painful Wrist

Carpal tunnel syndrome usually affects the hand Yin meridians (Heart, Pericardium and Lung). It can also affect the hand Shaoyang (Sanjiao) and very occasionally the hand Taiyang (Small Intestine) meridians. It often causes referred pain into the hand affecting all the fingers and the thumb.

Wrist pain includes pain as a result of a sprain, sports injury or more chronic and degenerative joint pain caused by arthritis, rheumatism or tendinitis.

Each treatment can be amended or modified for each specific case.

Once again a number of prescription options are suggested starting with the most comprehensive treatment that will address underlying deficiencies of the Kidney, Lung or, in the case of tendinitis, the Liver.

Option 1

Prescription for the Treatment of Carpal Tunnel Syndrome:

- Ren 12 (Zhongwan);
- Kid 17 (Shangqu) on the opposite side to move Qi from the Kidneys through the affected arm down to the wrist and the fingers;
- Then needle the shoulder point, St 24 (Huaroumen), Ab 1 (elbow) and Ab 2 (wrist) points on the affected side;
- If the pain radiates to the thumb use thumb point (Ab 3) and/or Ahshi points in this region;
- Finger Ahshi points will be found lateral to and between the level of the wrist Ab 2 and the elbow point Ab 1 These points should be located within a 0.5 cun proximity of these points. These Ahshi

points should only require very superficial needling to achieve the desired goal;

- Isolate the Ahshi points that best address the area of pain. They should be within a 0.5cun radius of the wrist (Ab 2) point. The depth variance for wrist conditions is minimal, and so it is best to rely on feedback from your client as to what depth cures the problem. As you move towards the extremities the depth is more superficial (see chapter 9, *Putting it all Together*, and case histories, 'A Drummers Wrist' and 'Simon the Shoplifter's Encounter with Security');

- A number of Ahshi points in the relevant areas will demand multiple needle formats such as a line, triangle or plum blossom to eradicate the radiating pain from the trapped median nerve (see Fig 8.10).

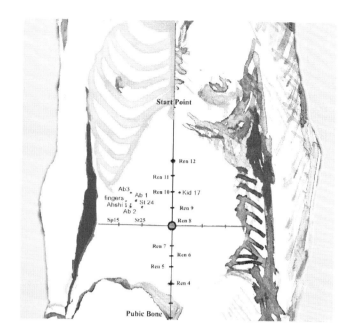

Fig 8.10. Prescription for carpal tunnel wrist pain to the digits

Option 2

Prescription for the Treatment of Wrist Pain due to Arthritis / Bi Syndrome

As described above for elbow problems, when there is an element of Dampness causing arthritic or rheumatic pain it is advisable to include the Feng Shi Dian (upper rheumatism points) also. If there is a degenerative condition, such as arthritis, a more comprehensive treatment is necessary.

You may choose to use 'Bringing Qi Home' or simply use 'Heaven and Earth' as described below. If there is Qi Stagnation, it is recommended that you include Ren 6 (Qihai) to move Qi.

- Ren 12 (Zhongwan);
- Ren 4 (Guanyuan);
- Kid 17 (Shangqu) contra-laterally;
- Then needle shoulder point, St 24 (Huaroumen) on the affected side;
- Needle the Feng Shi Dian combination to resolve the Dampness, Ab 1 elbow (upper rheumatism point) and Ab 2 wrist (upper lateral rheumatism point). These should be needled to a depth of 0.5 – 0.75cun;
- Isolate and treat the Ahshi points in the locality of the wrist Ab 2. Use three-star line or other formats as appropriate. Ahshi points at the wrist area will be quite superficial and the needles will probably be falling over as a result (depending on the area of the wrist being treated (See Fig 8.11).

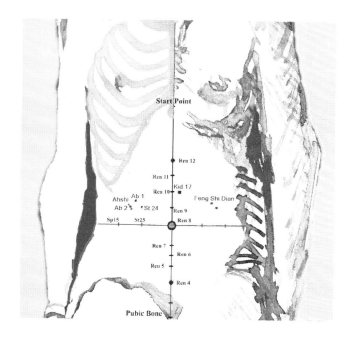

Fig 8.11. AA Prescription for wrist pain due to Bi Syndrome.

CASE STUDY: Simon the Shoplifter's Encounter with Security

Simon had a very limp and painful right wrist as a result of being restrained by means of a wrist lock by two security guards after his fourth attempt at walking out the back door of a large department store with a shopping trolley full of 42" plasma screen TVs! The previous three attempts had obviously been more fruitful for Simon! He was unable to lift his wrist unaided and, therefore, could not drive his motorbike and earn a living legitimately!

Simon was a heroin addict and this episode had led him to look seriously at what his drug addiction was doing to his life.

Treatment started with the Kidney and Spleen invigorating prescription of 'Bringing Qi Home' Ren 12 (Zhongwan), 10 (Xiawan), Ren 6 (Qihai) and Ren 4 (Guanyuan). As a lifetime of drug abuse had seriously depleted Simon, this combination was supplemented with bilateral Kidney 13 (Qixue). All three of which were placed to a depth of approximately 1 cun to strengthen the Kidneys. St 25 (Tianshu) was used bilaterally and Kidney 17 (Shangqu) on the left was needled to move Qi to the right arm. St 24 (Huaroumen) Ab1 (elbow) and Ab2 (wrist) were also penetrated with a triangular format used to break down the Ahshi nodes in the wrist area.

Upon enquiry Simon informed me that the pain in the wrist had reduced considerably from a reference point of 10 at the start to a more acceptable level of 4. With some fine adjustments of the needles in the wrist area the pain reduced to a level of 1 (see Fig 8.12). Traditional acupuncture points SJ 5 (Neiguan) and GB 34 (Yanglingquan) were used also to help locally and to nourish the ligaments. Additionally they helped ease Liver Qi Stagnation and calm a much-stressed body.

Simon left feeling much better and on his second visit he reported that his movement and pain in the wrist was definitely better. Treatment was repeated using the same prescription for a further four sessions by which time the wrist had improved enough to allow Simon to drive his motorbike.

He continued to have acupuncture for a number of weeks as he came off drugs and, as the wrist improved, the treatments changed to address his drug withdrawal issues.

Four years later and Simon is now fully recovered and off drugs. He is now working to rehabilitate other people afflicted with addictions. His wrist has not caused him any problems since, and he now pays for all of his shopping!

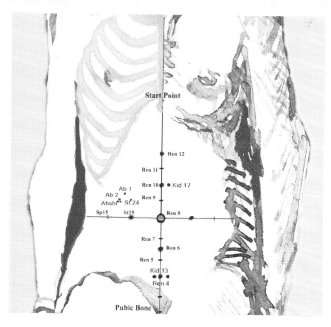

Fig 8.12. AA Prescription for 'Simon the Shoplifter.'

CASE STUDY: Drummer's Wrists

George, a 40-year-old professional drummer, was suffering with severe wrist pain. Affecting all six hand meridians, the pain was intense after a lot of use. George was also plastering his house and so the pain had become quite unbearable. He had been for traditional acupuncture before and decided to try abdominal acupuncture as he heard it was very powerful and he had a busy drumming season coming up.

Only two treatments were necessary and the prescription used was the same for both sessions. Ren 12 (Zhongwan), Ren 10 (Xiawan), Ren 6 (Qihai) and Ren 4 (Guanyuan) ('Bringing Qi Home') was used along with Kidney 17 (Shangqu) either side of Ren 10 (Xiawan). These were used contra-laterally to move Qi from the Kidneys through the shoulder and down both arms. Points Ab 1 (elbow) and Ab 2 (wrist) were also needled to enhance the movement of Qi down the arm to the wrists. Multiple Ahshi points were used on each side and 4-5 needles were used on each side in a diamond or plum blossom format (see, chapter 7, *Prescriptions: What's the Point*.) to cover the whole wrist where the pain was focused (see Fig 8.13). The depth of the needles varied from 0.1-0.3 cun and was dependent on results as expressed by the changes in George's pain levels.

George reported a huge improvement one week after the first treatment and he was surprised that he was able to continue with the labour intensive plastering work he had undertaken on his house. The second treatment used the same prescription as above although the depths may have changed slightly at the wrist points as the condition improved. On George's third and final treatment, a more minimal approach was used. Bilaterally Ab 2 (wrist) points were needled with two Ahshi points to give a triangular format in the area.

Two years later George is still drumming and has no problems with his wrists.

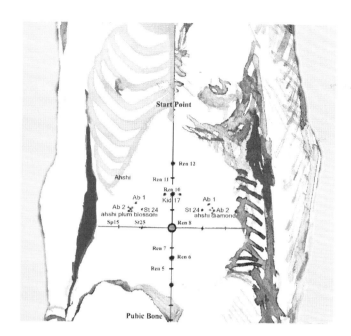

Start Point

Ren 12

Ahshi   Ren 11

Ren 10
Ab 1   Kid 17   Ab 1
Ab 2   •St 24   St 24 •   Ab 2
ahshi plum blossom   ahshi diamond
Sp15   St25   Ren 8

Ren 7
Ren 6
Ren 5

Pubic Bone

Fig 8.13. AA Prescription for case 'Drummers Wrists'

Pain in the Fingers and Thumbs

Treating finger and thumb problems is really a progression from the above and is best addressed using case histories. Where the condition has a deeper underlying causative factor, it will be necessary to use a comprehensive approach as is shown above with the 'Treatment of Wrist Pain due to Arthritis / Bi Syndrome'. Otherwise a minimal approach such as that used in the case study, 'Tom's Thumb', can be used.

CASE STUDY: Massage Finger

As a 38-year-old massage therapist, Martin was very worried about a cyst-like growth on his right index finger at the first phalangeal joint. The lump was the size of a pea and was painful after giving a massage. Martin had no other complaints other than a muzzy head in the morning and loose stools every day. His energy was good but often dipped in the afternoon. His tongue was scalloped and the pulse was full and soggy!

On investigation the abdomen was firm though it had some very small nodules either side of the umbilicus and also at Ren 9 (Shuifen). When palpating the area of the fingers just lateral and slightly distal to the wrist point (Ab 2), there was an obvious node the size of half a grain of rice! There was also a soft but palpable node at the left elbow point (Ab 1) at a deeper level indicating Spleen Dampness. The treatment would focus on clearing Dampness and removing the Phlegm from the hand area.

The prescription used was 'Bringing Qi Home', Ren 12 (Zhongwan), 10 (Xiawan), 6 (Qihai) and 4 (Guanyuan). This combination supplements the post-heaven with pre-heaven Qi and strengthens the Kidneys, Spleen and the Stomach. Kid 17 (Shangqu) was needled on the opposite side (left) to move Qi down the shoulder and through the entire right arm. The shoulder St 24 (Huaroumen), elbow (Ab 1) and wrist (Ab 2) were all needled to the heaven level. The finger area was needled with a triangular formation with the Ahshi point at the apex. This point was needled aggressively until the stubborn node had ceased to resist. To further reduce the Dampness the Sp Qi point (Ab 1) on the left was needled. In all, 12 needles were used (see Fig 8.14).

On checking with Martin, the pain only dissipated after the third Ahshi point was inserted and passed through the node. Martin took two weeks holiday from work and during this time he had four treatments. The same protocol was used with the number of Ahshi points reduced to one after the third treatment. The cyst on his palm was reduced dramatically within that fortnight and with two more treatments once a week the cyst disappeared completely. There was no more pain, even after a busy day of giving massage treatments.

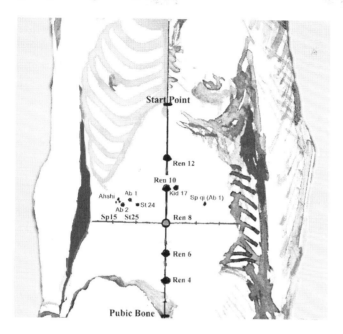

Fig 8.14. AA Prescription for case 'Massage Finger'

CASE STUDY: Tom's Thumb

A very worried graphic designer named Tom presented himself at the clinic complaining of severe pain around the thumb joint and moving along the Lung (Hand Tai Yin) meridian to the tip of the thumb. The main area of discomfort was around the thenar eminence and could be felt on the palmar and dorsal side affecting the hand Yangming meridian between LI 4 (Hegu) and around to Lu 9 (Taiyuan). The pain had started about two weeks previously and was progressively getting worse.

I suggested Tom focus on the areas of concern and explained how he should give each area a reference pain level of 100% of what it was at that very moment. I encouraged him to move the thumb to aggravate the pain to give a realistic idea of the pain.

The treatment used was minimal as he really didn't like the idea of acupuncture. 'Heaven and Earth' Ren 12 (Zhongwan) and Ren 4 (Guanyuan) was used with Ab 2 (wrist) and Ab 3 (thumb) on the right. On enquiry, the pain was no longer travelling to the tip of the thumb and had reduced slightly around the thenar eminence. I used two Ahshi points approximately 2 fen distal to the wrist points - and the depths were slightly deeper - to address the pain along the hand Yangming (LI) area, and a little more superficial to treat the hand Tai Yin (Lung) area of pain. The depths of the needles in these areas ranged from 1-3 fen (see Fig 8.15).

Once again I checked with Tom as to how his thumb was and he told me that the pain had disappeared, even with movement.

Tom returned for two more sessions and, following the initial treatment, the pain had only returned after overuse. Six months later the pain has not returned.

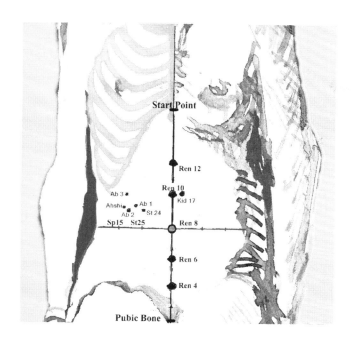

Fig 8.15. AA Prescription for case 'Tom's Thumb'

******Section Three******

Mid Back Rib and Chest Pain

When treating the mid back, it is important to remember the landmarks on the turtle hologram. Ren 9 (Shuifen) is level with thoracic vertebrae number seven (T-7) while Ren 8 (Shenque) is level with T-10 and Ren 7 (Yinjiao) is level with T-12.

CASE STUDY: Maddening Mastitis

Maria was a 39-year-old first-time mother of a seven-week-old baby, who was struggling against-all-odds to breastfeed. She developed painful lumps on her right breast and not recognising the signs let it become a painful infection for which she was treated with antibiotics two weeks previously. Maria was determined not to let this occur again and sought acupuncture as a means to this end. She was familiar with abdominal acupuncture and was delighted that it would not involve any needles near her affected breast.

Maria had a difficult birth and haemorrhaged heavily afterwards. For this reason it was decided to use 'Bringing Qi Home' with bilateral Kidney 13 (Qixue) to re-enforce the action of Ren 4 (Guanyuan) of nourishing the Kidneys. Points along the Kidney Meridian, level with Ren 9 (Shuifen), served a number of functions depending on the depth. Ren 9 (Shuifen) is level with thoracic vertebrae no 7 (T-7). The needle depth was initially left at 0.4-0.5 cun to nourish Blood by stimulating UB 17 (Geshu), the influential point of Blood, for approximately 20 minutes. These points are also level with the breast area and, in order to act on the chest area, the right needles were withdrawn to a more superficial depth of 0.1-0.2 cun for the remaining 20 minutes of treatment. Ren 9 (Shuifen) was also needled to help reduce the swelling of the breast. Ahshi points were located medially and inferior to St 24 (Huaroumen) on the right and these were needled superficially until all the nodes were dissolved and Maria's pain was gone. A four needle diamond pattern was used to achieve this (see Fig 8.16).

After the first treatment the pain and discomfort had reduced by approximately 50%, and she was advised to line her bra with raw cabbage leaves (they act as an anti-inflammatory). She had three more sessions using the same protocol, and the mastitis was cleared.

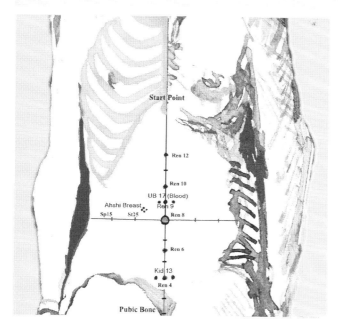

Fig 8.16 AA Prescription for case 'Maddening Mastitis'

******Section Four******

In this section we will cover how to treat all kinds of lumbar pain, from simple lumbago to more complicated sciatica with referred lower limb pain.

Treating Lumbar Pain

If it is an acute case, always needle Ren 9 (Shuifen) to reduce swelling. Ren 9 (Shuifen) is very helpful when there is a herniated or slipped disc. It is not necessary or beneficial to use this point with chronic backache. If the backache is chronic and the muscles are weak Sp 15 (Daheng) will help to nourish and strengthen them.

Option 1:

Treating Lumbar Pain

Start with 'Bringing Qi Home / Bringing Qi to the Source' i.e. points

Ren 12 (Zhongwan), Ren 10 (Xiawan), Ren 6 (Qihai) and Ren 4 (Guanyuan).

The function of 'Guiding Qi Home' is to supplement the pre-heaven Qi of the Kidneys with the post-heaven Qi and so invigorate the Kidney and Spleen to benefit the back. A person with a strong constitution will not require these points to be used when treating lower backache and sciatica (see minimal approaches below).

St 25 (Tianshu) will serve to relieve any mid-back spasm and relaxes the large latissimus dorsi muscles of the back. St 25 (Tianshu) may be used bilaterally or on the affected side only.

Use the point Ab 7 (Qipang) which is located along the Kid meridian on the opposite side to the affected leg, to move Qi from the Kidney to the affected limb. Qipang (Ab 7) can also act on the sacrum and lumbar area of the back.

Ahshi points are often felt as pea-sized nodes. These will usually be felt in the area (as represented on the hologram of the turtle) that anatomically represents the location of most pain, e.g. with hip or buttock pain Ahshi points should be in the area of St 26 (Wailing). When or if the needle encounters resistance at an Ahshi point, push through the resistance to break up the node and then pull the needle back to the original or required depth where pain relief is achieved (see chapter 6, *Abdominal Acupuncture Treatment Protocols* and chapter 9, *Putting it all Together*).

Needle St 26 (Wailing) on the affected side for one-sided low back pain or bilaterally if the pain is across the whole lumbar region. If this is a recurring problem use St 26 (Wailing) bilaterally as it will strengthen and relax the lumbar muscles, including the quadratus lumborum, longissimus and gluteus minimus, middimis, and maximus muscles. Look for the Ahshi points that best address the problem in this area and adjust the needle depth or add needles to rectify problems at different depths.

When the pain is located between L-1 and L-4 or L-5, feel for Ahshi points between Ren 6 (Qihai) and Ren 4 (Guanyuan). If the pain is more towards L-5 or the coccyx, you may have to check for Ahshi points between Ren 4 (Guanyuan) and Ren 3 (Zhongji).

If the problem is the result of a chronic condition, then it is likely there is some form of Kidney Vacuity and, therefore, it is recommended that points Kid 13 (Qixue) be used to tonify the Kidneys. These points will also serve to strengthen the related area of the back along the UB meridian in the region of UB 25 (Dachangshu).

If the pain is along the Huato Jiaji line on either side of the spine then you will find Ahshi points around the relevant vertebra line approximately 0.2 cun lateral to the Ren Mai. When there is pain along the UB meridian check on the Kidney meridian for anomalies that reflect the area of most discomfort and treat accordingly.

When the pain is in a line or covers a large area, a number of needles may be needed to address this. The needle formats used may resemble any of the previously mentioned formats such as a triangle, or if the pain is in a line, then the three star format should reflect this (see Fig 8.17). It is important to needle the most painful Ahshi (or the toughest node) first check the therapeutic outcome of this needle with your client, i.e. is the pain reduced or gone. If not, use that as the start point of the relevant format, i.e. if using a triangle, the first needle should be at the apex.

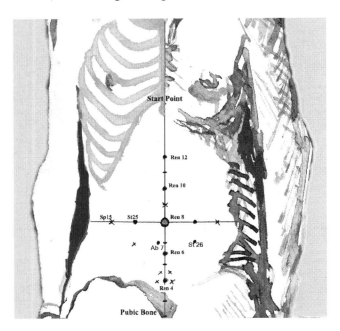

Fig 8.17. AA Prescription for treating Lumbar pain X's indicate possible points or Ahshi points to use depending on the nature of the condition

Option 2

A Little Bit of Minimalism for Lumbar Pain

If the client is young or of a strong constitution with no other underlying root cause for the lumbar pain, you may not need to use Ren 6 (Qihai) and Ren 4 (Guanyuan). Instead, use Spleen 15 (Daheng) bilaterally.

If the condition is acute use Ren 9 (Shuifen) to stop swelling and inflammation. Locate and treat Ahshi points as described above (see Fig 8.18).

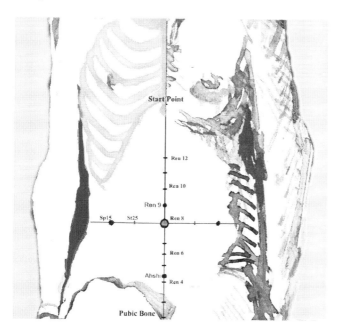

Fig 8.18. AA Prescription for Treating Lumbar Pain Option 2

Option 3

A little Bit More Minimalism for Lumbar Pain

You can always try the first treatment that Professor Zhiyun Bo used way back in 1972 to treat sciatica:

- Ren 6 (Qihai) and Ren 4 (Guanyuan);
- Locate and treat Ahshi points as described above (see Fig 8.19).

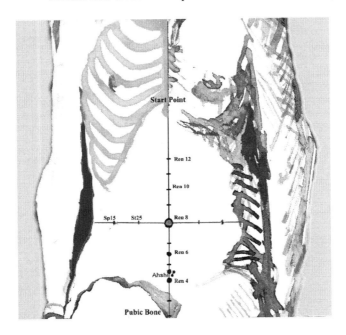

Fig 8.19. AA Prescription for Treating Lumbar Pain Option 3

Option 4

For Lumbar / all over back pain

- The 4 gates St 24 (Huaroumen) and St 26 (Wailing), combined with the prescription 'Regulating Spleen Qi', and Sp 15 (Daheng) bilaterally can be used to treat back pain where there is not a vertebra problem (see Fig 8.20).

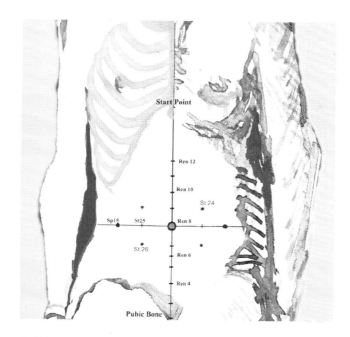

Fig 8.20. AA another prescription for treating lumbar pain

CASE STUDY: Sneezed and Seized (Acute Back Spasm)

Simon attended my clinic after he injured his back during weight training. The following day he had sneezed and his back completely seized up. It took him over an hour to get into a comfortable position where he was able to apply a heat pack and gradually get a little mobility into his back once again. He explained that the pain was mainly on the left side around UB25 (Dachangshu) and was radiating into his buttock with severe pain at GB 30 (Huantiao).

Points Ren 9 (Shuifen), Ren 6 (Qihai) and Ren 4 (Guanyuan) were needled. Ren 9 (Shuifen) was chosen because this point serves to reduce swelling in acute conditions. Kid 13 (Qixue) was chosen on the affected side to act as an Ahshi point and, because of the Biao Li relationship to the Kid meridian, can treat the UB. This location corresponds with the location of UB 25 (Dachangshu). St 26 (Wailing) the hip point was needled to a depth of (0.4 cun) at the heaven level to treat the pain at GB 30 (Huantiao). Sp 15 (Daheng) was needled bilaterally to nourish the muscles in the back and relieve pain and spasm. The pain was completely gone and free movement restored after only one treatment that only involved seven needles in total (see Fig 8.21).

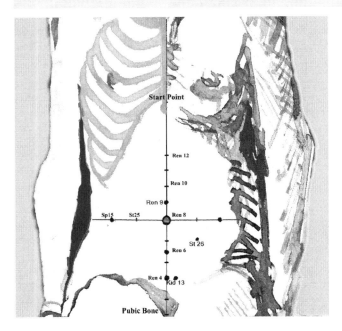

Fig 8.21 AA Prescription for case 'Sneezed and seized.'

Sciatic Nerves

Prescriptions for the Treatment of Sciatic Pain, with Referred Pain Moving Down the Leg to the Knee.

Option 1

Use the same protocol as with option 1 above for treating lumbar pain. If it is of an acute nature, then use Ren 9 (Shuifen) as described above.

If the pain is only on one side:

- Ren 12 (Zhongwan), Ren 10 (Xiawan), Ren 6 (Qihai) and Ren 4 (Guanyuan);
- St 25 (Tianshu) bilaterally or just on the affected side (I usually do bilaterally on the first or second visits; it will help to re-align the back);
- Ab 7 (Qipang) on the opposite side. This opens the gate to move Qi down the opposite leg;
- St 26 (Wailing) the hip point on the affected side;
- The Knee point (Ab 4) and ankle point (Ab 6) should be treated if the pain moves down the leg (only on the affected side) (see Fig 8.22).

> **Tip:** I often complete the circuit to move Qi down the whole leg on the first and second sessions as this type of referred sciatic pain often changes and moves further down the leg.

With all the main needles inserted to a superficial level, start to adjust each one to the correct depth, move from the top to the bottom. Correct the back pain first and then add Ahshi points or adjust depth of needles as required to get the best results;

When the pain is located on the medial aspect of knee, feel for Ahshi points between the knee point (Ab 4) and the medial knee point (Ab 5), which is located 1 cun medial to the knee point (Ab 4);

Use whatever needle format best addresses the area and the shape of the Ahshi points that reflect the pain;

Adjust the needle depths as necessary to stop the pain.

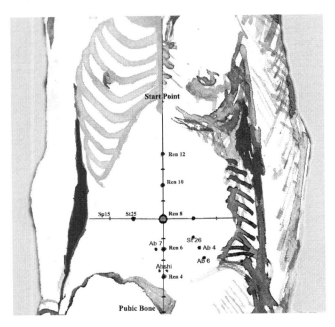

Fig 8.22. AA Prescription for treating sciatica with referred pain.

Option 2

A Little Bit of Minimalism for Sciatica with Referred Knee Pain Moving Down the Leg to the Knee.

Providing there are no other serious symptoms or deep-rooted causes, this more simple prescription will give effective results.

- Ren 6 (Qihai) and Ren 4 (Guanyuan);
- Use Spleen 15 (Daheng) bilaterally;
- If the condition is acute use Ren 9 (Shuifen) to stop swelling and inflammation;
- Ab 7 (Qipang) on the opposite side. Open the gate to move Qi down the affected leg;
- St 26 (Wailing) hip point on the affected side;
- With all the main needles inserted to a superficial level, start to adjust each one to the correct depth, move from the top to the bottom. Correct the lower back pain first before focusing on the leg;
- Locate and treat Ahshi points in and around knee point (Ab 4) and medial knee (Ab 5). Use whatever format to address the Ahshi points, area and size. For example, it may be necessary to put a line of needles between St 26 (Wailing), the hip point, and the knee point (Ab 4). When the pain is travelling in a line down the UB or GB meridian of the leg to the knee, use Ab 6 (Ankle) on first and/or second treatment;
- Adjust the needle depths and fine tune as above for best results (see Fig 8.23).

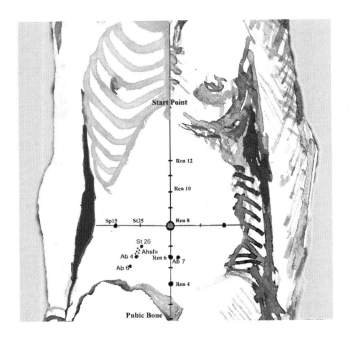

Fig 8.23. AA Prescription for treating sciatica with referred pain

Option 3

A little Bit More Minimalism for Sciatica with Referred Knee Pain.

Where there are no other symptoms or deep-rooted causes for the pain:

- Locate Ahshi points between Ren 6 (Qihai) and Ren 4 (Guanyuan), including any points between Ab 7 (Qipang) and down to Kid 13 (Qixue), that best reflect the anatomical area of pain as reflected by the hologram of the turtle;

- Locate and treat Ahshi points in and around the knee point (Ab 4) and medial knee (Ab 5). Use whatever format necessary to best address the general nature and size of the Ahshi points;

~ 252 ~

- Adjust the needle depths and fine tune as described above for the best results (see Fig 8.24).

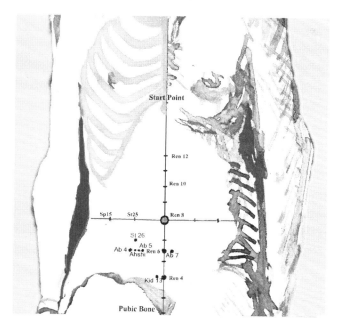

Fig 8.24. AA Prescription for treating sciatica with referred pain.

Prescriptions to Treat Sciatica with Referred Pain Moving Down the Leg to the Ankle:

Low back pain with referred pain down to the ankle is more than likely due to putting pressure on the sciatic nerve. This can be verified by a leg raise test.

The prescription to use in this case is the same as the first treatment for lumbar pain with referred pain moving down the leg to the knee (see Fig 8.22).

Once all the needles have been inserted, and the low back pain is resolved, then your attention should move to the ankle pain.

In the case of ankle pain, find Ahshi points around Ab 6 (ankle point) on the affected side and as described above. Adjust the needle depth and location as appropriate and remember that the depth will be more superficial as you move down towards the extremities.

CASE STUDY: A Dancer's Potential Disaster (Acute Low Back Pain and Sciatica)

Sarah hurt her back during rehearsals on the morning of the opening night of a very physically demanding six-week show. She complained of severe pain around lumbar vertebra no.4 (L-4) with radiating pain down the right foot Tai Yang (UB) meridian to UB 57 (Chengshan). She could not move let alone dance. Treatment was conducted on the floor of the rehearsal studio as Sarah was in so much pain and was very concerned about her back, but she was determined that 'the show must go on'.

The original treatment prescription was points Ren 12 (Zhongwan), Ren 9 (Shuifen), Ren 6 (Qihai) and Ren 4 (Guanyuan). Ren 9 (Shuifen) was used to reduce swelling in this acute case of sciatica. Kid 13 (Qixue) was chosen on the affected side to act as an Ahshi point and, because of the Biao Li relationship between the Kidney and the Urinary Bladder (UB) meridian, this location corresponds with the location of UB 25. Qipang (Ab 7) was punctured on the left to move Qi through the right leg. St 26 (Wailing), the hip point was needled deeper (0.4 cun) at the heaven level to treat the pain at GB 30 (Huantiao). Ab 4 (knee point) was inserted to a depth of 0.2-0.3 cun and Ab 6 (ankle point) completed the circuit to move Qi down the entire affected limb. An Ahshi point was located midway between Ab 4 (knee) and Ab 6 (ankle), which reflected the painful area of UB 57 (Chengshan) where Sarah's pain terminated in a severe fashion. Sp 15 (Daheng) was needled bilaterally to nourish the muscles in the back and relieve pain and spasm there (see Fig 8.25).

Sarah's pain disappeared within five minutes of starting the treatment, and she was able to stand up straight and walk without any pain after the 45-minute session. She performed a very physical show that night and went on to complete the six-week run of the show with only a couple of follow-on treatments.

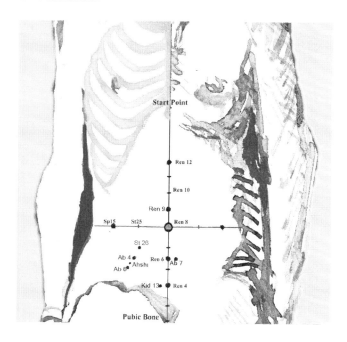

Fig 8.25. AA Prescription for 'A Dancer' Potential Disaster'

CASE STUDY: Dick's Herniated Disc

Dick, a 29-year-old golf enthusiast, had injured his back at the driving range. He had a herniated disc between his fourth and fifth lumbar vertebrae (L-4 and L-5) more than eight months previously and had decided to try acupuncture on a friend's recommendation. He had severe pain that was concentrated mainly on the right side of his lower back UB 25 (Dachangshu) and into his buttock along the GB channel at GB30 (Huantiao). The pain was radiating down his right leg along the UB meridian, and the worst pain was in the region of UB 62 (Shenmai), which he described as feeling like a hot poker being stuck into the bone.

Dick had to cancel three holidays due to his pain and the depression he was suffering was as a result. When he attended a specialist he was told that the only option was surgery. That was a terrifying concept for Dick and left him feeling fearful and depressed. He had attended a physiotherapist who had helped to a degree, but he felt that he had achieved as much relief through this route as he was going to get.

Dick read about the work I was doing with abdominal acupuncture and explained that he was prepared to give it a try for as long as it would take to make his pain go away. He was asked to use a reference score of 10 out of 10 on the pain as it was at that very moment in each of the different areas.

1. Low back
2. Buttock GB30 (Huantiao)
3. Calf UB 57 (Chengshan)
4. Ankle UB 62 (Shenmai)

Treatment began with abdominal acupuncture and the points chosen were as Follows: (See Fig 8.26).

A combination of 'Bringing Qi Home' Ren 12 (Zhongwan), Ren 10 (Xiawan), Ren 6 (Qihai) and Ren 4 (Guanyuan) was used to strengthen the Kidneys and Yuan Qi, and nourish Marrow. It also serves to strengthen all of the back;

Sp 15 (Daheng) bilaterally to ease pain and spasm in the back. It also serves to nourish the muscles that had been suffering over the 8 months;

St 26 (Wailing) bilaterally to nourish and ease pain in the lower back. On the right hip two Ahshi points were used at depths ranging from 0.3-0.5 cun to address the pain in the buttock area;

Kid 13 (Qixue) was needled bilaterally to treat the herniated disc at L4-L5. An Ahshi point between Ren 4 (Guanyuan) and Kid 13 (Qixue) on the right was also used to treat along the Huato Jiaji line on the back;

Ab 7 (Qipang) was used on the left to move Qi from the Kidney through the right leg;

Ab 4 (knee) and Ab 6 (ankle) were needled and Ahshi points midway between these were used slightly more superficially to stop the pain in the calf. Ab 6 (ankle) had a number of Ahshi points which formed a diamond structure and these points reduced the burning sensation and halved the pain in the area of UB 62 (Shenmai).

As the treatment proceeded Dick's pain eased in all areas to a comfortable 2 or 3 on a score of 1-10. The ankle area was a bit more stubborn and the pain reduction there was approximately 50%.

Dick returned two days later and he reported that the pain had remained at a reduced level, but that the ankle was still extremely painful, after long periods of sitting. Treatment continued with the same main prescription on the abdomen (see Fig 8.26). A particularly resistant nodule around the ankle area required 3 needles in a triangular format at the ankle with the main Ahshi point located at the apex of the triangle. The pain relief was more impressive this time with a reduction to a very comfortable score of 2 down from 10. The calf pain was no longer a major issue and the lower back pain was also reduced.

I consolidated the treatment with traditional acupuncture including SI 3 (Houxi) on the left and UB 62 (Shenmai) on the right. GB 34 (Yanglingquan) was also used on the right. On his next visit, Dick reported that he was able to travel home (a one hour journey) standing on the train without any pain and felt that the same pain relief was equivalent to the relief felt if he had taken *Diaphene*. This was the first time he had a pain free journey home in over eight months. His mood was improving and he was beginning to see a light at the end of this long tunnel!

In the fourth and fifth session the treatment continued primarily with abdominal acupuncture. Progress continued and Dick then took a 4-day trip to Italy where he did up to four hours walking on one day. His ankle pain was aggravated and once again abdominal acupuncture was combined with some mirror imaging (Tan, R. 2007, pp 35-42) left Ahshi point around Lu 9 (Taiyuan), to address the severe ankle pain. On this occasion the nodule at the ankle position Ab 6 was extremely tough to break through at the superficial depth of approximately 0.2 cun. The needle eventually passed through the node and it was broken down using vigorous manipulation and then returned to a depth of 0.2 cun. The relief once again was very impressive at 80%.

During the seventh session Dick reported that he had little pain in the back or calf, the ankle pain was down by 80%, and he had even forgotten about it on occasion. His mood had improved and he was planning his next trip abroad.

Treatments were then reduced to one per week, and there was continuous progress with the ankle area remaining the only focal point for pain. Dick had a total of 14 sessions and when he finished he only had occasional ankle pain on cold days or after overuse. The pain he experienced was down to a level 2, i.e. an 80% reduction of what it had originally been.

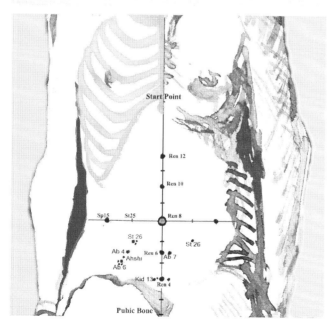

Fig 8.26. AA Prescription for treating case 'Dick's Herniated Disc'.

CASE STUDY: Driven to Drugs (Sciatica)

Andrea was a recovering heroin addict who had severe sciatic pain that was preventing her from driving and made walking extremely difficult. The pain radiated down to her buttock around GB 30 (Huantiao) and often moved down her right leg. On the first visit she explained that the pain was due to a slipped disc and that she was scheduled to have surgery in the next few weeks. She didn't know what the surgery would entail and didn't really care as long as it got rid of the pain. She expressed her concern that this pain was going to drive her to use heroin again, the thoughts of which were giving her nightmares.

Treatment given was intended to nourish the pre- and postnatal Qi with the 'Guiding Qi Home' format of Ren 12 (Zhongwan), Ren 10 (Xiawan), Ren 6 (Qihai) and Ren 4 (Guanyuan). Kid 13 (Qixue) was used bilaterally to reinforce Ren 4 (Guanyuan) and treat the lumbar vertebra 4 (L-4) area of pain. Sp 15 (Daheng) was used to ease the spasm in the back. St 26 (Wailing) was needled bilaterally to strengthen the lower back and stop the pain at GB 30 (Huantiao). Three Ahshi point needles were used in a line on the right side. Even though this was a chronic problem, it was decided to use Ren 9 (Shuifen) because of the slipped disc, and the area felt a little lumpy so intuition told me to try it on this occasion. (See Fig 8.27). Andrea reported that her pain had eased substantially to a dull ache.

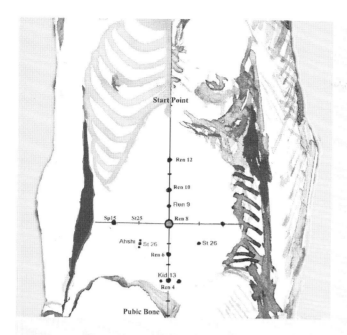

Labels visible in figure:
Start Point
Ren 12
Ren 10
Ren 9
Sp15   St25   Ren 8
Ahshi   St 26   ● St 26
Ren 6
Kid 13
Ren 4
Pubic Bone

Fig 8.27 AA Prescription for treating case 'Driven to Drugs'.

After the first session she was able to drive her car and was confident that she could beat this without relapsing back to using heroin. She had less pain but as the days went by between her weekly treatments the pain returned.

On her second visit the pain was travelling down her right leg along the Tai Yang Urinary Bladder (UB) meridian as far as UB 40 (Weizhong) where the pain was quite intense. The treatment again used 'Bringing Qi Home' with Kid 13 (Qixue). This time Ren 9 (Shuifen) was not used. There were some small nodules between the Kidney and Ren meridians on the right just above the level of Ren 4 (Guanyuan). These were needled as they reflected Huato Jiaji points around L-4 where the disc problem was located. On this occasion St 25 (Tianshu) and St 26 (Wailing) were also needled on the right (the affected side) to ease pain and spasm of the lumbar area.

(Qipang) Ab 7 was used on the left side and St 26 (Wailing) on the right was used to move Qi down the right leg. (Ab 4), the knee point, was needled to a depth of approximately 0.3-0.4 cun until the pain at UB 40 (Weizhong) was gone. Three needles were used in a triangular form to give maximum relief (see Fig 8.28). Andrea was able to drive her car once more after this treatment.

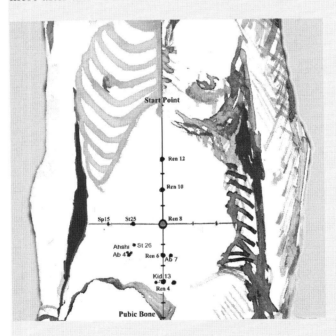

Fig 8.28. AA Prescription for treating case 'Driven to Drugs'.

Surgery was postponed as Andrea had a flu, which gave her the opportunity to have two more abdominal treatments. Both sessions focused on strengthening the back to correct the misaligned disc at L-4 and stop pain at UB 40 (Weizhong) using the same protocol as the earlier second session.

I didn't see Andrea again for eighteen months when she returned after injuring her back while putting clothes in the washing machine. She told me that she had the surgery and that the doctors commented that they had expected the surgery to take a lot longer than it did. She added that they were surprised the condition was not as serious as previously thought.

******Section five******

Abdominal Acupuncture Prescriptions to Treat Lower Limb Problems

- Knee pain;
- Ankle problems, such as sprained ankle;
- Foot conditions such as plantar fasciitis;
- Toes, including neuralgia.

In order to prevent repetition, it is possible to treat most of these in a similar way as they were treated for sciatica with referred pain moving down the leg to the knee or ankle, as noted above. Obviously it will not be necessary to use Ahshi points to treat lumbar pain.

If there are other factors involved in any of the above conditions, such as arthritis or other type of Bi Syndrome, then a more comprehensive treatment is needed. Tailor the prescription as your diagnosis dictates, i.e. if there is Bi Syndrome with Dampness affecting the lower aspect of the body use the lower Feng Shi Dian points, Ab 4 (lower rheumatism point) and Ab 6 (lower lateral rheumatism point) bilaterally. The below case

histories, 'A Needy Knee' and 'Degeneration of Knee Cartilage at 23',
give a comprehensive account of how to treat knee problems.

CASE STUDY: A Needy Knee

Annabel was a 58-year-old office worker who walked a number of miles
to and from work at a good pace every day. She enjoyed walking.
However, having previously had knee problems with her other leg, she
contacted me with a crucial ligament problem that was keeping her awake
at night and preventing her from walking any distance even at a slow pace.
She suffered from anxiety and worried about the implications of the knee
problem.

Her abdomen was warm above and cool and clammy below the navel.
There was a definite solid node between the area of points Ab 4 (knee) and
Ab 5 (medial knee) on the affected right side. The exact area of pain on the
medial aspect of her knee was located and marked with iodine to monitor
changes in pain as the acupuncture proceeded. Upon pressing this area
Annabelle was asked to take note of the intensity of the pain and to give it
a reference point score of 10.

The first treatment used the 'Guiding Qi Home' to supplement Spleen and
Kidney Qi, along with just the knee point where the nodule was
prominent, i.e. the medial knee (Ab 5). This point was difficult to
penetrate past 0.1 cun and the needle had to be rotated vigorously in order
to get through the resistance enforced by the nodule. After needling
through the node more rotation was used to diminish the node and relieve
pain. Upon achieving a reduction to the resistance, the needle was left at a
depth that gave the best pain relief, i.e. 0.1-0.2 cun (see Fig 8.29).

On the second visit, Annabel reported a significant improvement in the pain at night but claimed that walking still caused some pain. The same prescription was used and the knee point (Ab 4) was added as there was now some pain from the front of the knee around St 35 (Dubi). Palpation indicated that the original nodule had reduced in size. The abdomen still felt a little clammy below the navel. Her tongue was also scalloped with a white coat and her pulse was slippery. With all these indications of Dampness, it was decided to add Sp 15 (Daheng) to invigorate the Spleen function, nourish and lubricate the joints and expel Dampness. In all eight needles were used.

On the third visit there was no more pain from the front of the knee and the medial pain was reduced. However, when walking there was still an awareness and a fear of walking at a brisk pace. Overall Annabel reported that her energy levels were better and that her sleep was good.

On this occasion it was decided to use the following more comprehensive prescription of 'Bringing Qi Home' Ren 12 (Zhongwan), Ren 10 (Xiawan), Ren 6 (Qihai) and Ren 4 (Guanyuan). This combination has a general tonifying effect and was good for Annabel's general constitution, for as a 58-year-old woman it was helpful to nurture the Kidneys Yuan Qi. Ab 7 Qipang was used on the contralateral side to capitalise on the Kidney Qi and to move it from the source to the afflicted right knee. St 26 (Wailing) the hip point was punctured in order to move Yangming Qi down the right leg. The lower rheumatism points, i.e. Ab 4 (knee) and Ab 6 (ankle), were needled bilaterally to expel Wind and Dampness from the lower limbs.

The needle depths at the arthritic points were superficial initially on the right side to treat the affected knee pain and then were put to a depth of 0.5 cun after 15 minutes to act at a deeper level and clear the Wind and Dampness. An Ahshi point that reflected the medial knee weakness was needled between the Ab 4 and Ab 5 points (See Fig 8.30). St 26 (Wailing) was left at a superficial level throughout. On the last visit this prescription was repeated and Annabel reported more confidence walking since the pain had not returned. As a result, her level of anxiety had decreased also.

It is important to be flexible with your treatments and sometimes there is a need to focus a little more on the causative factor (Dampness) in order to get longer term results. Adjusting the depth of the needles can have a profound effect on the therapeutic result so be prepared to adjust the depth of the needles during individual treatments and throughout the course of therapy as a person's condition changes.

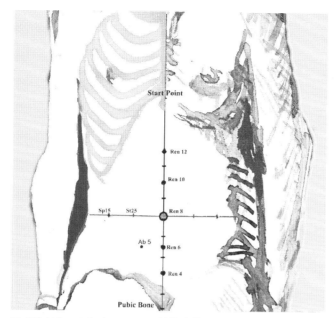

Fig 8.29. AA Prescription for treating case 'A Needy Knee'.

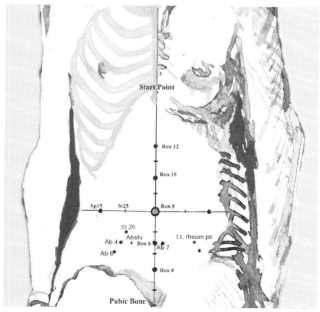

Fig 8.30. AA Prescription for treating case 'A Needy Knee'

CASE STUDY: Degeneration of Knee Cartilage at 23

Tom, a 23-year-old sportsman, had to stop playing Gaelic football because of his severe knee pain. He continued to play hurling but had to take a number of weeks off to try and repair the degenerated knee cartilage with acupuncture. Tom had already had two surgeries on his right knee and one on his left over the past ten years since his knee problems had begun. He was eager to avoid more surgeries as the time scale of his pain relief was less following each operation.

Tom was healthy and enthusiastic and was prepared to work at repairing the damage to his knees. He was in severe pain following a match and experienced a lot of tightness all around his knees and radiating up into his thighs along the Spleen, Liver and Gallbladder meridians. We agreed on a treatment plan that would entail two treatments per week and include refraining from hurling training for two weeks.

For the first session of abdominal acupuncture the prescription used was Ren 12 (Zhongwan), Ren 6 (Qihai) and Ren 4 (Guanyuan), with Qipang (Ab 7) being used bilaterally to enable Qi to move from the Kidneys down both legs. The prescription was then completed by using bilateral hip points St 26 (Wailing), knee points (Ab 4) and ankle points (Ab 6). All points were inserted superficially initially, and needle depths were then fixed to the correct levels.

Upon enquiry Tom reported that the left knee pain and leg tightness was gone and that the right leg still had some tightness, primarily along the Gallbladder and Spleen meridians. There was still some pain on the lateral aspect of the knee and slightly superior medially around Sp 10 (Xuehai).

Palpation at the initial investigation of the abdomen had revealed some nodes around the whole of the knee. These points were investigated again and some Ahshi points were isolated around the knee points (Ab 4) and medial knee (Ab 5) (see Fig 8.31). At this stage I enquired as to the level of pain in each of the areas. There was only one area of discomfort left that was above the knee at Sp 10 (Xuehai) on the right side. One more needle was inserted slightly medial to and superior to the knee point (Ab 4). This was at a superficial level of approximately 0.2cun. In total, there were four needles used in the area to correct the problem and the depth of these ranged from 0.2-0.4 cun.

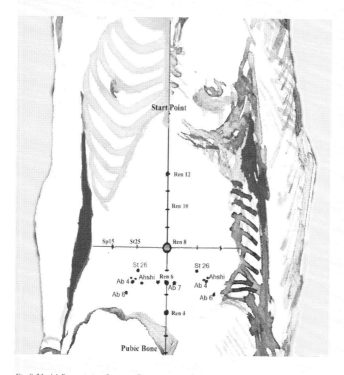

Fig 8.31. AA Prescription for case 'Degeneration of Knee at 23'

Tom was amazed at the speed and accuracy of the treatment and was relieved to think that there was a real alternative to knee surgery.

Tom returned three days later and reported that he had almost no pain or tightness in his left leg and that the right side was approximately 50% better than it had been.

Treatment continued along the same lines as previously, and the right leg was once again pain-free. I continued to treat the left leg to ensure that the results would be long term and because I was aware that Tom would be back playing competitive sport in less than two weeks.

On the third visit Tom acknowledged that 'he had not felt so good since just after his first knee surgery!' The prescription used on this occasion was very minimal and only the knee points on both sides were used. Two needles on the left relieved the very slight tightness while three on the right relieved the 20% pain (compared to his first visit) that was there. Tom was delighted that his reference point score of 10 as measured when he arrived for the third treatment had now gone down to zero. I decided to add Sp 15 (Daheng) bilaterally to assist with nourishing the muscles and to lubricate the joints (see Fig 8.32).

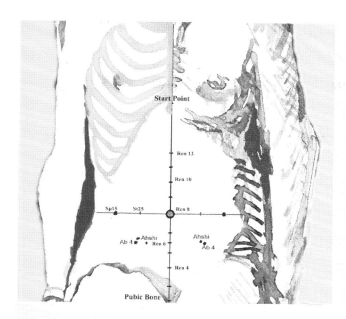

Fig 8.32 AA Prescription for case 'Degeneration of Knee at 23'

On the next visit Tom reported that he had done some light training and played a friendly match and following this, he had no pain on the left and very slight discomfort with some tightness on the right. Tom was delighted with the result and was confident that his future in competitive sport was looking much brighter.

Over the next four sessions the focus was on the right knee and treatments alternated between minimal and more comprehensive treatments as described above.

Tom returned to full-contact hurling matches, and he had no pain on either leg. He had some tightness around the knee following one particularly demanding game that was relieved by some gentle massage by the team physiotherapist.

Three months later and Tom is still enjoying his renewed vigour on the hurling pitch.

Abdominal Acupuncture Prescriptions to Treat a Sprained Ankle / Ankle Injury

An ankle injury such as a sprain is often very painful and usually involves a lot of swelling in the area. This is the case with many such sudden injuries, and it is usually advisable to avoid the area in question and to use distal points or some form of imaging such as abdominal acupuncture (abdominal acupuncture has many advantages over other forms as described in the advantages of AA in the introduction to the book).

Option 1

Prescription to treat a sprained or injured ankle

At the acute phase use Ren 9 (Shuifen) to reduce swelling. It is also advisable to use Sp 15 (Daheng) if there is severe pain accompanying the inflammation.

- Ren 12 (Zhongwan);
- Ren 9 (Shuifen);
- Ren 6 (Qihai) * This will resolve Qi Stagnation and so it should be used where there is Qi Stagnation;
- Ren 4 (Guanyuan);
- Ab 7 Qipang contralaterally;
- St 26 (Wailing) hip point, Ab 4 (knee) and Ab 6 ankle points on the affected side;

- Find Ahshi points around Ab 6 (ankle point) on the affected side and adjust the needle depth and location as appropriate. Use the number of needles that best cures the pain in any of the formats, such as plum blossom, etc. Remember that the depth will be more superficial as you move down towards the extremities (see Fig 8.33).

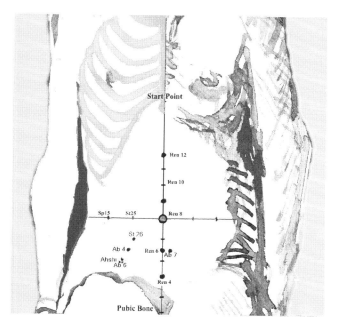

Fig 8.33. AA Prescription for treating sprained or injured ankle.

Option 2

<u>A More Minimal Prescription to Treat a Sprained / Injured Ankle:</u>

- Ren 6 (Qihai). This will resolve Qi Stagnation and so it should be used where there is Qi Stagnation;
- Ren 4 (Guanyuan). This will assist in moving Blood Stasis;

- Find Ahshi points around Ab 6 (ankle point) on the affected side and adjust the needle depth and location as appropriate. Use the number of needles that best stops the pain in any of the formats such as triangular, three star or diamond structure etc (see Fig. 8.34).

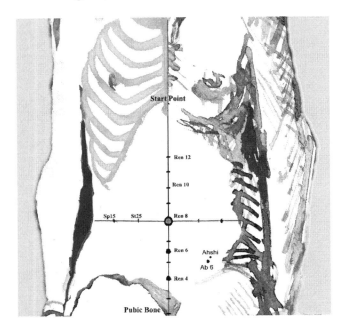

Fig 8.34. AA Prescription for treating sprained or injured ankle

The treatment of feet and toes is best highlighted with case histories. It is similar to the above ankle prescription with the addition of Ahshi points to locate exact areas of pain. You will notice that I often use St 27 (Daju) when treating feet and toes as it is anatomically equivalent to the location of Kidney 1 (Yongquan). I have found that using St 27 (Daju) will give the best results if they have not been achieved without it.

CASE STUDY: Diabetic Happy Feet (Neuralgia due to diabetes)

Bernie, a 70-year-old heavy drinker and smoker, was attending the clinic with sciatica, which was causing her severe pain down the right foot Tai Yang and Shaoyang (UB and GB) meridians. The pain was along the UB meridian to UB 40 (Weizhong) and was most intense at GB 30 (Huantiao). After a few treatments Bernie mentioned that she hadn't been able to put the bed sheets over her feet for a year or so due to neuralgia in her feet as a result of her diabetes. She had been told that her feet would more than likely have to be amputated in the next 12-18 months.

Treatment focused on moving Qi through both legs and into her feet using the following prescription. The underlying aim was to nourish the pre- and postnatal Qi with the 'Guiding Qi Home' format of Ren 12 (Zhongwan), Ren 10 (Xiawan), Ren 6 (Qihai) and Ren 4 (Guanyuan). St 25 (Tianshu) as the front Mu point of the Large Intestine was used bilaterally to clear Excess Heat and to strengthen the mid back area. It also helps to move Qi from the Yangming meridian which has copious Qi. Ab 7 (Qipang) was needled bilaterally to direct Qi through the contralateral lower limb. St 26 (Wailing), the hip point, was punctured to a depth of approximately 0.4 cun on the right to ease pain in the buttock area of GB 30 (Huantiao). On the left it remained at a depth of approximately 0.2-0.3 cun. Ab 4 (knee pt.) and Ab 6 (ankle pt.) were needled more superficially and foot Ahshi points were located and, when not obvious to touch, were located using the blueprint of the turtle, i.e. around 0.5-1.0 cun below and 0.5 cun medial to the ankle points (see Fig.8.35). Three needles were inserted on either side to cover the toes. One treatment made a dramatic difference and on the next visit Bernie was delighted to declare that she was able to sleep with the bed sheets covering her feet. A further five treatments were given, and the neuralgia was no longer a problem for Bernie. One year later there was no re-occurrence and Bernie was happy to have both of her feet still attached!

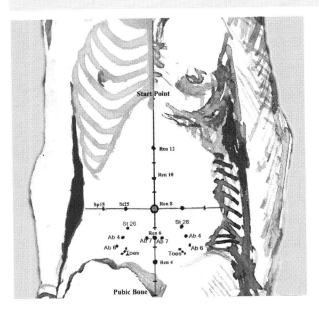

Fig 8.35. AA Prescription for treating case 'Diabetic Happy Feet'

CASE STUDY: The Fabulous Flipper Foot (Loss of Strength and Sensation in the Feet)

Michael reluctantly came for acupuncture on the advice of his brother. He was 52 years old, and his work was very physical and mostly outdoors. Michael had fractured his fourth and fifth lumbar vertebra (L-4 and L-5) when he was in his mid-30s and was lucky enough to make a full recovery. He had experienced bouts of sciatica over the years and, after a particularly bad episode affecting both left and right foot Tai Yang (Urinary Bladder) meridians, he had been left with his two feet feeling like they were 'flippers'. He described this feeling as a weakness that left him unable to stand on his toes, and he had to give up playing tag rugby as a result. His back was not causing him any pain, and there were no other symptoms.

Michael was strong and fit in all other respects, and he had learned how to deal with the episodes of pain, but this weakness and foreign body feeling was very disturbing to him. He was a 'no bullshit' type of guy and was a bit perplexed by the concept of having needles put in his stomach when his problem was with his feet! I assured him that this was the best approach and, as he was very reluctant to have acupuncture for his previous bouts of sciatica, I sold abdominal acupunctures merits by highlighting the fact of minimal needle sensation with maximum therapeutic effects!

With Michael's history, the 'Guiding Qi Home' supplemented with St 25 (Tianshu), St 26 (Wailing) and St 27 (Daju) bilaterally. The points Ab 7 Qipang were needled bilaterally to open the gate and allow Qi move from the Kidneys through the lower limbs. Knee (Ab 4) and ankle (Ab 6) points were punctured bilaterally to complete the hip (St 26 Wailing), knee and ankle circuit and allow Qi to flow completely down the leg and into the foot. St 27 (Daju) was chosen as it is equivalent to the Kid 1(Yongquan) point on the sole (See Fig 8.36). At the end of the treatment Michael was surprised that his feet felt, in his words, 'more real'.

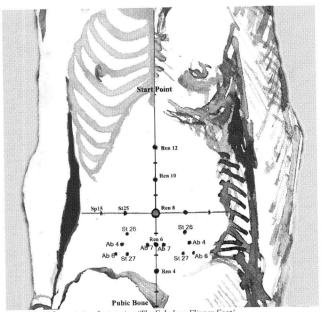

Fig 8.36. AA Prescription for treating 'The Fabulous Flipper Foot'

He returned the following week and reported that he was much calmer and less stressed than normal even though he was going through a difficult time with his business. He was more open on this occasion and told me that he had also experienced some headaches in the last three months. He was happy that his feet were becoming more responsive and were feeling less 'alien'.

I repeated the same prescription and added the right elbow (Ab1) point to calm the Liver. I also added Kid 13 (Qixue) bilaterally to support the Kidney Essence so that it would nourish the Liver Essence also and benefit both the headaches and the numbness of the feet. On his next visit he was very upbeat and happy that he had not had any more headaches, and his feet were becoming stronger.

Michael had two further treatments and made a full recovery. He returned to playing tag rugby, and his feet remain functional parts of his body to this day!

CASE STUDY: Twinkle Toes that had lost their Sparkle (Toe Pain)

Tina's toes had lost their sparkle and at the age of 55 she often had pain in both the first and second metatarsals. The pain was difficult to describe but often stopped her from enjoying long walks and frequently forced her to sit down rather than dance at concerts. There was a constant numbness and 'foreign body' feeling from her toes and the top of her foot. This strange feeling could turn to pain when the surface under foot was ridged, such as in the shower. Tina was also experiencing broken sleep due to night sweats and was menopausal.

On the first three treatments the prescription used was 'Guiding Qi Home', Ren 12 (Zhongwan), Ren 10 (Xiawan) and Ren 6 (Qihai), and Ren 4 (Guanyuan) to nourish the Kidneys and Spleen, which were clearly Vacuous. Kidney 13 (Qixue) was also needled bilaterally to support and further nourish the Kidney Essence. Ab 7 (Qipang) was needled bilaterally to direct Qi through the opposite leg and into the feet. St 26 (Wailing) the hip point and was punctured to a depth of approximately 0.2-0.3 cun. Ab 4 (knee pt.) and Ab 6 (ankle pt.) were needled more superficially. Foot Ahshi points were located and, when not obvious to the touch, were located using the blueprint of the turtle, i.e. around 0.5-1.0 cun below and 0.5 cun medial to the ankle points (see Fig.8.37). Three needles were inserted on either side to cover the offending toes. St 27 (Daju) was also needled bilaterally because it is in the location of Kid 1 (Yongquan) and has a strong tonifying effect on the Kidneys, and, from my experience, has a great influence on correcting problems with the feet.

Tina's strange sensation and the discomfort was progressively reduced following the first few sessions. Her sleep had also improved, and she was no longer disturbed by night sweats.

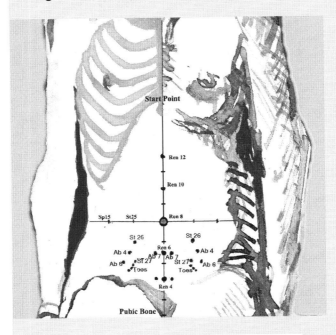

Fig 8.37. AA Prescription for treating case 'Twinkle Toes that had lost their Sparkle'.

The next five sessions used the prescription of 'Heaven and Earth' Ren 12 (Zhongwan) and Ren 4 (Guanyuan). This combination was enough to support the Kidneys, and Kid 13 (Qixue) was no longer deemed necessary. The remainder of the treatments were varied and points alternated so that for session two and four, only points St 27 (Daju) and the Ahshi points around the toes were used (see Fig. 8.38). On sessions one, three and five, points Ab 7 (Qipang), St 26 (Wailing), Ab 4 (knee) and Ab 6 (ankle) were

~ 280 ~

needled also. The result was that Tina had fewer episodes of pain, and the degree of numbness or alien-like feeling, decreased to a much more tolerable level.

Tina was able to enjoy a three-day music festival where standing didn't cause any major discomfort.

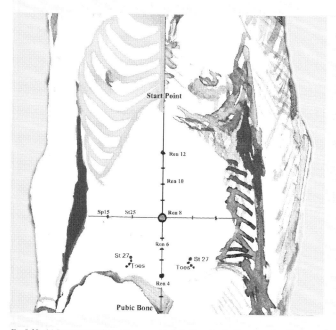

Fig 8.38. AA Prescription for treating case 'Twinkle Toes that had lost their Sparkle'

******Section Six******

Abdominal Acupuncture Prescriptions for Hip Pain

Option 1

If the hip pain is of a chronic nature a comprehensive treatment to address the Bone and joint is recommended.

Start with 'Bringing Qi Home / Bringing Qi to the Source', i.e. points.

- Ren 12 (Zhongwan), Ren 10 (Xiawan), Ren 6 (Qihai) and Ren 4 (Guanyuan);
- St 26 (Wailing) will serve to move Qi to the greater area of the hip. It may be used bilaterally or on the affected side only;
- Where there is some form of Kidney Vacuity, it is recommended that points Kid 13 (Qixue) be used to further tonify the Kidneys. These points will also serve to strengthen the related area of the back along the UB meridian in the region of UB 25 (Dachangshu).

When treating hip pain feel for any Ahshi points around St 26 (Wailing) on the affected side. Needle depth should reflect the depth of the hip pain. Needle around the area until the pain has reduced, adjusting the depth as necessary. Use whatever needle format best treats the general nature of the reflected Ahshi points (see Fig 8.39). If the hip pain is covering a large anterior area - for example, from GB 29 (Juliao) to St 31(Biguan) - a needle format such as the plum blossom or diamond format may be necessary to fully address the whole area of discomfort. The needle depth will be more superficial than if the pain was more to the posterior hip region.

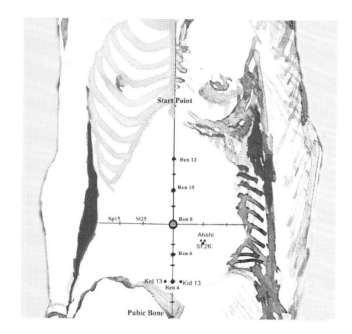

Fig 8.39. AA Prescription for Treating Hip Pain

Option 2

Abdominal Acupuncture Prescriptions for Hip Pain - A Little Bit of Minimalism:

When the hip pain is not due to an underlying chronic Deficiency type, it is possible to simply use points below the umbilicus. If the pain is of an acute nature use Ren 9 (Shuifen) to reduce inflammation.

- Start with Ren 6 (Qihai) and Ren 4 (Guanyuan);
- Locate and treat Ahshi points in and around the hip point St 26 (Wailing) and use whatever format to address the Ahshi points, area and size. For example, it may be necessary to put a triangular or **Y** type format in the vicinity of St 26 (Wailing);

~ 283 ~

- Adjust the needle depths and fine tune as above for best results;
- If the pain is originating from the sacrum use Ab 7 (Qipang) on the affected side to treat this area (see Fig. 8.40).

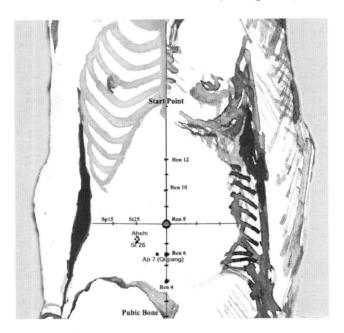

Fig 8.40 AA Prescription for treating hip pain

Option 3

Abdominal Acupuncture Prescriptions for Hip Pain - A Little Bit More Minimalism:

Providing your client has no other causative factors or symptoms it is possible to treat hip problems with just Ahshi points.

- Locate and treat points in and around the hip point St 26 (Wailing) and use the best needle format to address the Ahshi points, area and size. For example it may be necessary to put a triangular or **Y** type format in the vicinity of St 26 (Wailing):

- Adjust the needle depths and fine tune as above for best results.

CASE STUDY: A Gangster's Hip

Tony, a 60-year-old ex-con and former enforcer for a now extinct but once notorious Dublin criminal gang, came to me suffering from severe hip pain located at GB 29 (Juliao). The pain was stabbing in nature and was stopping him from his martial arts training and preventing him working as a doorman.

He had tried one session of acupuncture in a busy franchise acupuncture chain and found that the local needles were too painful and that they aggravated his already debilitating pain.

We discussed our options and decided to use a minimal abdominal approach and then, if needs be, build on that in later treatments. I was very aware that he was suspicious of acupuncture and had only come to me on a trusted friend's recommendation.

Tony had no problem putting a pain score of 10 on his hip and he only had to lift his leg to feel the severe stabbing pain. Palpation of the area revealed a pea-sized node around St 26 (Wailing), at a fairly superficial level. It was obvious that the cause of the pain was due to Blood Stasis and so it was important to move Blood.

Treatment started with 'Heaven and Earth', i.e. Ren 12 (Zhongwan) and Ren 4 (Guanyuan), and was supplemented with Ren 6 to move Qi and thus assist the function of Ren 4 (Guanyuan) in moving Blood. After needling St 26 (Wailing) to a depth of 0.3 cun on the affected right side, I checked how the pain had changed. The intensity and area of pain had changed, and I added two more Ahshi points slightly lateral in a superior and inferior manner to give a triangular format (see Fig. 8.41). These points were also at a similar depth, and once again I enquired as to the level and location of the pain. At this stage it had dramatically improved, and a very slight reduction of depth on the Ahshi points gave a more comprehensive reduction in the overall pain.

Tony was visibly impressed and shared his enthusiasm for this treatment as opposed to the other acupuncture he had received. I saw Tony twice more over the next four weeks, and he was able to return to work as a doorman, which involved long hours standing outside a nightclub in Dublin's cold and wet winter nights. On the third visit he reported that the pain was almost completely gone, and he decided that he was going to return to his martial arts training. However, he would be sure to contact me if the hip acted up again. I have not heard from him three years later.

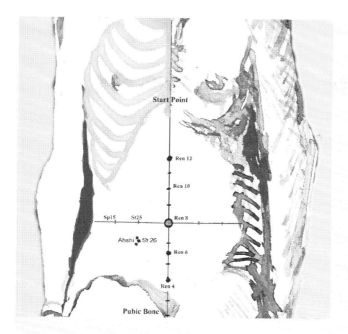

Fig 8.41. AA Prescription for treating case 'A Gangsters Hip'

****

Less is Not Always More! A Few Words on Minimalism

When you first start using abdominal acupuncture, I strongly recommend that you use the first or second option prescriptions suggested above. These prescriptions have been tried and tested and have proved to be consistently effective. As you develop and become more self-assured with your abdominal palpation, accurately locate Ahshi points, you will become more confident with what depth is necessary to get the best result. When you have been steadily getting good results then you can start to explore using fewer needles.

In my experience I have found that when treating a pain in the limbs - for example, an ankle or elbow pain - better results are achieved by using the whole limb treatment with the contralateral Kidney point to move Qi from the Kidney to that limb (see above), than if the affected area was treated on its own.

A client who had pain on both wrists came for treatment and on the first session just the wrist points were used with three needles on each side quite superficially to relieve the pain completely. The pain returned the next day and pain was radiating up her forearm at times. Because the results obtained were only short-lived on the next three sessions both shoulder, elbow and wrist points were used after using Kid 17 (Shangqu) bilaterally to move Qi through the arms. The results achieved were long lasting and comprehensive. On other occasions I alternate treatments so that the whole limb is treated on one day and only Ahshi points in the area affected are used on alternate treatments. This method gives better results than when only Ahshi points are used.

******Section Seven******

A Final Complicated Case

CASE STUDY: Accident Prone Anita (Upper Back, Shoulder and Neck Pain Combined with Sciatica and Hip Pain)

Anita first attended my clinic as a result of severe debilitating back, neck, shoulder, arm and hip pain. Anita's first misfortune happened twenty years previously when she fell off a motorbike on holidays and was lucky not to end up in a wheelchair. Since then Anita had limited mobility in her neck and also experienced pain down both arms, particularly down her right arm. Twelve years later she had another accident skiing, which aggravated her original injuries.

Her latest incident happened when she slipped on ice while carrying a heavy camera causing her to break her right hip and collarbone. The camera was unscathed! As a result of the intense pain, Anita was not sleeping at night and had to quit her job. Initially, she was treated twice a week using points, as indicated on Fig 8.42. The prescription of 'Bringing Qi Home' i.e. Ren 12 (Zhongwan), Ren 10 (Xiawan), Ren 6 (Qihai) and Ren 4 (Guanyuan). Primarily this was used because of its strong tonifying effect on the Spleen and the Kidneys, Yuan Qi, and nourishment for the Marrow. Equally it also serves to strengthen all of the back which had been damaged at different stages of Anita's life.

St 25 (Tianshu) was needled bilaterally to help move Yangming Qi (in conjunction with St 24 (Huaroumen) and St 26 (Wailing) throughout the body), with the aim being to strengthen Anita's mid back. Kid 17 (Shangqu) was punctured bilaterally to move Qi from the Kidney and direct it into the upper limbs. Next, St 24 (Huaroumen) was inserted bilaterally and then Ab 1 (elbow) and Ab 2 (wrist) points were needled on each side. As her right hip was painful and both sides of her low back were stiff and often sore, St 26 (Wailing) was punctured bilaterally in order to reduce the stiffness and relieve the spasm in the back. With all three Stomach points listed above the all over back pain was being addressed.

Due to the fact that Anita's problems began twenty years previously it was also decided to use Kid 13 (Qixue) to strengthen the Kidney and treat the lower back pain. With all the needles in superficially they were adjusted to their correct depth starting with the Ren points. Following that was the

Kidney and finally the Stomach and Ab 1 (elbow) and Ab 2 (wrist) points. St 24 (Huaroumen) was needled to a depth of 0.2-0.3cun to address the front shoulder pain on the right.

Anita checked where the pain was and reported it was now more to the back, and another needle was inserted slightly deeper and this stopped the pain from GB 21 (Jianjing). The only remaining pain was at the base of her neck along the trapezius muscle. This was corrected by a slight increase in the depth of the right Kid 17 (Shangqu) needle (see Fig 8.42). All the other points were adjusted in a methodical way and the result checked either directly by gauging the change in pain or by the information received from each needle, i.e. whether the resistance at Ahshi points had reduced.

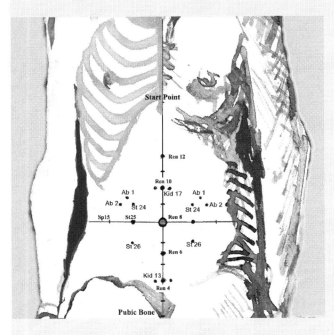

Fig 8.42. 'Accident Prone Anita' prescription one points

Her pain eased in her neck and upper back quickly and within a week the focus of the treatment was then directed towards her hip and right-sided sciatic pain.

The prescription used was 'Bringing Qi Home' with St 26 (Wailing) bilaterally due to the all-over low back pain and general weakness. To move Qi down the right leg, Ab 7 Qipang was used contra laterally. St 26 (Wailing) on the right had a triangular needle format to address the front, back and side hip pain and in order to facilitate this, the needles were placed at different depths ranging from 0.1-0.4 cun. As the sciatic pain was located between GB 30 (Huantiao) and UB 40 (Weizhong) needles were added at Ab 4 (knee) and Ab 6 (ankle) to correct the movement of Qi throughout the right leg (see Fig 8.43).

As Anita's condition improved the leg points were changed slightly, and the ankle point (Ab 6) was dropped in favour of a straight line format of four needles from the hip to the knee. These needles went to a depth of approximately 0.3 cun (see Fig 8.44).

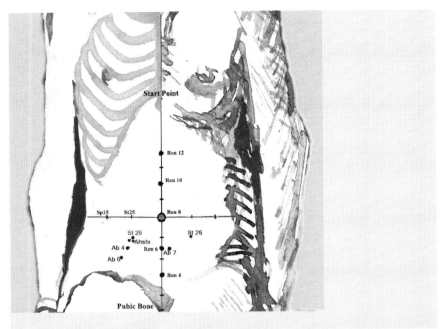

Fig 8.43. 'Accident Prone Anita' second prescription points

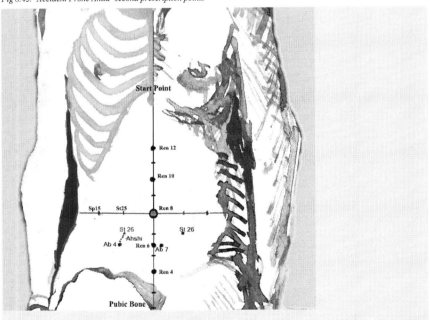

Fig 8.44. 'Accident Prone Anita's third prescription points

After six treatments the focus moved to treat the Damp Bi Syndrome, which had developed over the years. The prescription used was 'Bringing Qi Home' combined with upper (Ab 1) and upper lateral (Ab 2) rheumatism points, and lower rheumatism (Ab 4) and lower lateral (Ab 6) rheumatism points. The action of this combination would tonify the Kidneys and Spleen, thus strengthening the Bones and muscles, clear Dampness, stop pain and lubricate the joints (see Fig 8.45).

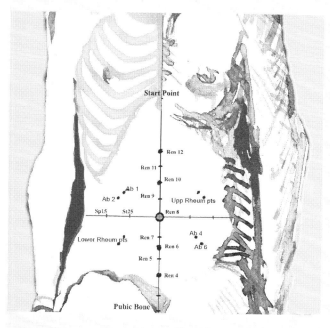

Fig 8.45. AA Prescription four 'Accident Prone Anita' - Bringing Qi Home & Feng Shi Dian

Anita's recovery continued at a staggering pace and within a short period she was able to sleep through the night and stop taking pain medication. She has since started her own knitting business and only occasionally had to return for treatment after a particularly busy week of knitting.

Conclusion to this Case

This case was complicated with pain affecting virtually the whole body. It highlights how AA can be used to treat a multitude of problems at the one time. Initially treatments involved a lot of needles to correct the all over body pain while also addressing the underlying Disharmonies that had arisen throughout the years. As treatments progressed, the focus moved to more specific areas such as the hip and sciatic pain. Then, with further improvement, the overall aim was to broaden the therapeutic action by treating the Damp Bi Syndrome and reduce the number of needles down to 12 from a maximum of 28! (See Figs 8.43 to 8.45.)

Anita's case highlights the importance of staying focused and systematic throughout the AA treatment. It is important to check with your client at relevant times, such as when adjusting or adding Ahshi needles, asking, 'How has that affected the pain in this particular location?' This information should be noted so that you have a full picture of exactly which needles are likely to have the best effect at each painful location.

Failure to gain this comprehensive view will result in you tweaking random needles in the hope that you choose the right one. Being precise at each stage will give you more credibility and by asking questions at the right time it will avoid you having to bombard your client with inaccurate questions that will frustrate patients and test their patience!

******Section Eight******

The Treatment of Headache and Sensory Problems

As with other conditions, the treatment of headaches, facial pain and sense organ problems can be done in a number of ways depending on the causative factors.

I am confident that, at this stage, you are probably able to pre-empt the possible treatments I could offer. So rather than spell them out for you I will give a few pointers as to the most important aspects to consider when treating the above conditions. I will use the following case histories to indicate this rationale!

CASE STUDY: A Total Headcase (Headaches)

One of the most impressive results I ever had came from a demonstration I gave. The client, John, had suffered a severe brain injury as a result of a shelf that was holding around 50 kgs of boxes on it falling and hitting him on the temple in a freak accident.

John had tried every painkilling medicine, medical and otherwise possible. None had given any real relief. The next option open to him was to have surgery to 'numb part of his brain', but this was only being offered in the USA, and he could not risk the flight as the change in air pressure could easily kill him in his current condition. John volunteered to be treated, and I explained to the audience that really this was a challenging case. His injuries left him in excruciating pain 24/7 from:

1. The left temple to the right temple;
2. Fengchi GB 20 on the right to Taiyang M-HN-9 (extra) on the left.

Treatment started with the commonly used prescription of 'Bringing Qi Home', Ren 12 (Zhongwan), Ren 10 (Xiawan), Ren 6 (Qihai) and Ren 4 (Guanyuan) in order to supplement the post-heaven with pre-heaven Qi, thus strengthen the Kidneys, Yuan Qi, and nourish the Marrow.

Upon palpation of the area above Ren 12 (Zhongwan) Ahshi points were located by the presence of small superficial knots. These Ahshi points were needled quite superficially (0.1-0.3 cun). Following this John reported his temple pain had reduced to a very comfortable score of 2 (down from 10). More Ahshi points were discovered between Ren 11 (Jianli) and Ren 12 (Zhongwan) relating to the pain covering the area from GB 20 (Fengchi) to Taiyang (M-HN-9). Once again following superficial needling the pain completely disappeared within seconds (see fig 8.46). (To my relief, as I wondered if I had bitten off more than I could chew with an audience watching!)

This treatment was done in a demonstration setting and was in the presence of some twenty observers. After a 30-minute treatment John reported that it had given him the best pain relief ever, noting that even opiates had not given such powerful relief.

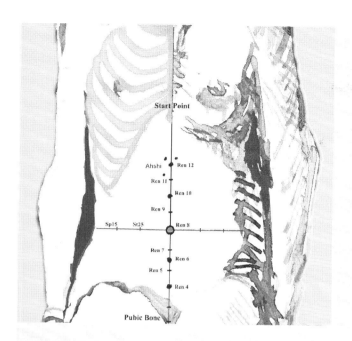

Fig 8.46. A Total Headcase Prescription

CASE STUDY: Headaches from Hell

Helen attended the clinic on the advice of her physician. Her physician had
made the suggestion knowing that Helen was not happy with the medical
alternative of a lifetime on anti-epilepsy drugs to control her 'new onset
daily chronic headaches'. Over a period of months she had developed
headaches that affected her along the foot Shao Yang (Gallbladder), the
foot Tai Yang (Urinary Bladder) and foot Yangming (Stomach)
meridians. The pain moved from front to back and often was more intense
around the forehead and behind the eyes. She often felt that her skin was
super sensitive and even light touch felt almost electric at times. The pain
was relentless, and it had impacted on her mood so much so that she burst

into tears while explaining her symptoms and the suggested western medical prognosis.

Helen had decided to take time off work running her busy restaurant. Family life had been very difficult in the preceding year with the death of a loved one and a family feud over the estate. Helen's periods had become very painful with clots and debilitating cramps on the first and second day of menstruation. Nothing seemed to ease the cramps and, as a result, she had to take strong painkillers and stay at home in bed on the first day of her cycle.

Helen's headaches were in various locations:
1. Temporal at extra point (M-HN-9) Taiyang;
2. Electric tingling sensation along the gallbladder meridian from GB 14 (Yangbai) through to GB 20 (Fengchi);
3. Stabbing pain behind the eyes.

Helen had a wiry and slightly rapid pulse. Palpation of her abdomen revealed a number of small bead-like nodes around and above Ren 12 (Zhongwan). She also had a node at the elbow point (Ab 1) (at the earth or Ba Gua layer) on the right which reflects the Liver area and specifically treats Liver Qi Stagnation. Ren 4 (Guanyuan) felt slightly weak. There were no discernible temperature differences. Treatment was aimed at moving Liver Qi Stagnation dredging the affected meridians and resolving the pain.

The prescription used was 'Bringing Qi Home', Ren 12 (Zhongwan), Ren 10 (Xiawan), Ren 6 (Qihai) and Ren 4 (Guanyuan). This would serve to strengthen the Spleen, Kidneys, Yuan Qi and Liver Essence, and nourish Marrow. Ahshi points above Ren 12 (Zhongwan), just lateral to the

Kidney meridian approximately mid-way between Kid 19 (Yindu) and Kid 20 (Futonggu), were needled to varying depths ranging from 0.1 cun to treat the frontal aspect and 0.3 cun to treat the back of the head. Ahshi points around Kid 19 (Yindu) were needled to a depth of approximately 0.2-0.3cun to address the discomfort at GB 20 (Fengchi). Special point Ab 1 (elbow) was used on the right to ease Liver Qi Stagnation. St 24 (Huaroumen) was punctured to move Qi through the Yangming meridian to the head. After all the needles were intially inserted they were put to their correct depth, and any nodes were broken down using a strong manipulation of the needles until they had become less resistant to penetration.

On enquiring, Helen reported that the headache had initially eased and then it seemed to move to just above the eyes. The electric sensation vanished and with the insertion of two more superficial needles near the Ahshi points above Ren 12 (Zhongwan) the pain eased to a very tolerable 2-3 from an excruciating level of 10 (see Fig 8.47).

Helen was initially treated twice a week, and her headaches had reduced in intensity and frequency following the first session by about fifty percent. Three more treatments were conducted using the same main prescription and only slight adjustment of Ahshi points were made as required. Helen reported a further decline in headaches. They were now occasional and didn't require medication.

After five treatments Helen was feeling more confident and returned to work for a busy weekend. She got a comparatively mild headache following two long shifts on her feet 'meeting and greeting' her customers.

The electric sensation was no longer evident and the headaches, when they did occur, were mainly temporal.

Helen had a further twelve treatments over three months, during which she has only had a couple of headaches brought on by extreme stress. The headaches were very mild and of a shorter duration in comparison to what she originally experienced.

Helen now has almost no PMS (pre-menstrual syndrome) symptoms. Her severe dysmenorrhoea, which had demanded she stay at home and take at least eight of the strongest codeine based painkillers on the first day of her cycle, now only required, at worst, two paracetamol (mild) painkillers and no longer required bed rest. Thus, Helen could continue with her busy life.

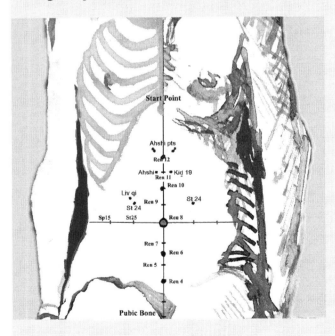

Fig 8.47. AA Prescription for treating case 'Headaches from Hell'

CASE STUDY: Tina with the Twitching Eye

Tina had been suffering with a twitch in her eye for over two months when she first came for acupuncture. She worked as an event organiser and had to spend a lot of time at a computer, her work tended to be intensive and stressful coming up to an event. The twitch had become constant and was more pronounced with stress and tiredness. Tina was healthy in all other aspects and the twitch was due to Wind in the Shaoyang meridians.

For the initial treatment I did not use abdominal acupuncture as Tina was menstruating and was feeling quite vulnerable about her abdominal area. Traditional acupuncture was used, and I choose to use local points including Yintang (M-HN-3) directed towards UB 1 (Jingming) of the affected eye. Taiyang (M-HN-9) on the affected side, GB 20 (Fengchi), San Jiao 5 (Waiguan) and Liv 3 (Taichong) were all needled bilaterally.

On her next visit Tina reported that the treatment had given some temporary relief in the first couple of days but that the twitch had returned with the same degree of seriousness as before. On this occasion it was decided to use abdominal acupuncture and the diamond prescription was used with Ren 12 (Zhongwan), Ren 4 (Guanyuan) and St 25 (Tianshu) bilaterally to nourish the Spleen and Kidney. I chose Ren 4 (Guanyuan) over Ren 6 (Qihai) as it is more influential on the Liver. Ab 1 on the right also known as the Liver Qi point was also needled. Upon palpation a very small but palpable node 0.3cun superior and to the right of Ren 12 (Zhongwan) was only needled to a depth of 0.1cun as it was working on the eye. Extra points to nourish the eye 1 cun lateral to and level with Ren

7 (Yinjiao) were needled bilaterally to a depth of approximately 0.5 cun to the level of Humanity (see Fig 8.48).

Conventional acupuncture continued to be used including SJ 5 (Waiguan) on the Right, Liv 3 bilaterally and Yintang (M-HN-3) directed towards the right UB 1 (Jingming). Following this treatment there were only two minor episodes of twitching and these occurred after long hours of intensive work at the computer. It was two weeks before Tina returned and on this visit the above prescription was repeated without using the eye Ahshi point. Six months later Tina's eyes were still sparkling without a twitch.

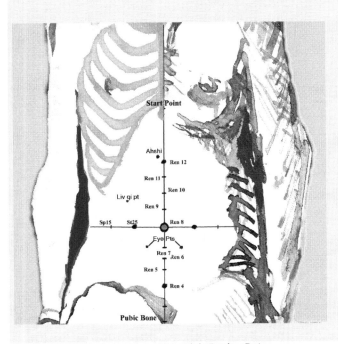

Fig 8.48. AA Prescription for treating case 'Tina with the Twitching Eye'

****** **Section nine** ******

Conclusion

All of these cases show the power of abdominal acupuncture. Often the prescription seems very similar for very different conditions. The same points may be used but the depths are often different thus giving very different results. In each case the importance of feedback from the client cannot be overestimated. In the few cases where results are not immediate, it is important to trust your intuition and be led by the evidence from palpation and the knowledge of what area reflects specific anatomical areas of the body as portrayed by the map of the turtle.

In many of the cases, although a lot of different symptoms are presenting at the same time, it is important to focus on the main areas of pain. Then, as these improve, maintain the focus on the areas of greatest pain or discomfort. By virtue of the general prescriptions, including the four Ren points of 'Bringing Qi Home,' the whole body is being strengthened and is, therefore, able to rectify disharmony.

Using minimal points, in my experience, can be done when the client is strong and the condition is more acute. Using only points that reflect the area of complaint, such as the shoulder, in these situations will often give long-term relief. In clients who have been suffering chronic shoulder pain, for example, it is best to use a more comprehensive treatment, such as that used in the case study, 'A Busy Chef's Neck and Shoulder Pain' in section 1, rather than the more minimal treatment used for the 'A Case of Frozen Shoulder' in section 2.

Keep good records (see Appendix Figs A1 to A6 for record charts) and after you have treated various conditions repeatedly, you can then start to experiment to find what works best for you and your clients.

Be prepared to be flexible with your treatments. Abdominal acupuncture points will vary so be fluid. Remember the map of the turtle should only serve as a guide and even within that map there are some different interpretations. In fact, some literature suggests that Ren 4 (Guanyuan) is at the level of the fifth lumbar vertebrae while others say it is at the level of the fourth vertebrae. Through my clinical experience and my Centreforce AA training courses, I find that Ren 6 (Qihai) treats the first vertebrae and that Ren 4 (Guanyuan) is more level with L-4. This means that L2 and L3 will be found between Ren 6 (Qihai) and Ren 4 (Guanyuan). This being the case you should still be fluid with your thinking and find the location that treats your client best using palpation of and feedback from your patients.

When I ran my first Centreforce AA training course, I was reluctant to use the hologram of the turtle as I had never had one in China. When I was taught AA, we used simple prescription diagrams in the form of a vertical and horizontal line (in the shape of a cross, just as I use for my prescriptions in the Appendix (Figs A1-A4) at the end of this book). With this simplistic approach, I found I never got hung up on particulars of where various body parts were on the map of the turtle.

I found the group that did my first class were fixed in locations of areas such as the fingers, toes and the vertebra, and it made it difficult to relay the idea of fluidity of the exact location of anatomical areas. This confusion was very valuable to me later on, but at the time I wanted to take the turtle and drop-kick it into the deepest ocean I could find! Please always keep your cup half empty - that way you can fit more in.

Summary of Topics Covered in this Chapter

Creating confidence in treating a whole range of conditions covered in each section.

➢ Section 1

Tailoring treatments to treat upper back and neck problems

➢ Section 2

Treat Conditions of the Shoulders, Upper Limbs and Digits

Including:

- Frozen shoulder/shoulder pain
- Shoulder and referred arm pain
- Tennis elbow
- Carpal tunnel syndrome/wrist pain
- Arthritis or Bi Syndrome, and all kinds of problems affecting the hands, fingers and thumbs, including repetitive strain injury (RSI)

➢ Section 3

Mid back, rib, breast and chest pain

➢ Section 4

Treatment of all kinds of lumbar pain

- lumbago
- sciatica with referred lower limb pain

➢ Section 5

Abdominal Acupuncture Prescriptions to Treat Lower Limb Problems

Including:

- Knee pain
- Ankle problems, such as sprained ankle
- Foot conditions such as plantar fasciitis
- Toes, including neuralgia

➢ Section 6

Abdominal acupuncture prescriptions for hip pain

➢ Section 7

- **Treating complicated cases**

➢ Section 8

- **The treatment of headache and sensory problems**

➢ Section 9

- **Conclusion and a word on minimalism**
- **Keeping your own prescription notes.**

Chapter 9: Putting it all Together

Learning Objectives

In this final chapter, we address how to put all the information together in a logical and simple way. You will learn how best to treat clients with abdominal acupuncture so that you get the best results possible from the start. You will also learn more about the subtleties of treating with abdominal acupuncture and how to improve your intuition and confidence with each treatment.

General Considerations

After you have taken your initial case history, be as methodical as possible so that you can treat each complaint or the most important of a number of complaints. Do this in the best way using the most efficient number of needles, given the nature of the problem/s and the timing of the treatment. By the 'nature of the problem' I am referring to whether it's an acute one-off condition or a long-term chronic issue. The timing of the treatment refers to whether this is the first treatment with abdominal acupuncture. If this is the case, then it is often better to be comprehensive with the treatment, and it will probably require that more needles are used than if it were the third or fourth treatment.

Questions for Guidance

Use the following topics to guide you through your treatment:

What's the problem?

What are you trying to treat?

Is this a chronic or an acute condition and if so how will this affect the treatment plan?

Is this a deep rooted Bi Syndrome problem with an element of Dampness, Wind, Heat or Cold and if so, how and what implications will this have for the overall treatment?

Where is the problem/pain?

The client might have pain in the lower back moving into the buttock and around to the front of the hip.

Where would you expect to find Ahshi points?

It is important to note where the pain seems to be originating and where the most painful points are. Remember that pain at the front of the hip will respond better to more superficial needling than pain at the back of the hip or in the buttock. In this case the most effective treatment will include a number of needles around the hip point St 26 (Wailing) at varying depths from 0.1 or 0.2 cun for the front area to 0.3-0.5 cun for the back. If the pain is also halfway down the thigh where would you expect this to be represented on the hologram of the turtle?

What is the Abdomen Telling You?

When investigating the abdomen of the client is there any more information to be gathered from the abdomen? A client presents with pain in the right shoulder. Upon palpation the area around St 24 (Huaroumen) on the right is cold to the touch. Will the client then respond well to local heat? Does your client have a constitutional Kidney weakness, which is indicated by a (relatively) short distance between the pubis synthis and Ren 8 (Shenque)? Or is there evidence of Kidney Yin and/or Yang Deficiency? Perhaps the client has a constitutionally weak Spleen as indicated by a belly button that protrudes? All these clues will lend to a more specific and comprehensive overall treatment for your client.

Make a reference score for each pain!

Encourage each client to tune into their pain (see chapter 6, *Abdominal Acupuncture Treatment Protocols*) as it is when they lie down, and put a score of 10 or 100% on each pain that they have at that very moment in time. If they need to move the affected limb or area of the body to gauge the pain, this can usually be done without any difficulty when using abdominal acupuncture.

Have your client move and locate the pain before treatment so that they have a realistic account of improvement following acupuncture. Alternatively if you can isolate the painful point and press on it to gauge the change in pain before treatment and again as you are fine tuning the needles use this method to indicate the improvement in pain scores.

In this way as a practitioner you begin to isolate the exact needle and the depth that gave the best result for each pain. Check with the client at each stage as to the impact of the treatment on the pain level at each area being treated. Once you have reduced the main area of pain by an acceptable level of 50-100%, then move on to treat the next most painful area, or work in a systematic way.

If there is pain in the hip, knee and ankle on the left side, and there is also pain on the right shoulder and wrist, then treat one limb at a time (after all of the main needles have been inserted). I usually work from top to bottom, i.e. upper limb first!

What if there is no pain at the present time?

Proceed with the treatment as normal as there should still be Ahshi points in the relevant area. Locate and treat these as normal and trust your intuition as to the depth and location that you would expect to get the best results.

Tip: Encourage your client on the day of treatment to avoid taking pain killing medication, if at all possible. This will give you more realistic and accurate feedback and leave no doubt in your client's mind as to where the pain relief is coming from.

What is the treatment plan?

Decide on the best treatment plan for the client. If it is an acute problem and there is local inflammation, Ren 9 (Shuifen) will relieve the spasm and inflammation. If there is Bi Syndrome with all over pain, it would be best to use the Feng Shi Dian combination to clear the Wind Damp in combination with 'Bringing Qi Home'.

Decide what is best for your client and formulate your prescription. If the patient reports better results from a more comprehensive treatment then continue with that. Often I will rotate treatments one day doing a full treatment using all points as prescribed above. Then on the next visit I will use the more minimal treatment as described in Chapter 8, *Abdominal Acupuncture Prescriptions for Frequently Seen Painful Conditions* section five, case history 'Twinkle Toes that had lost their Sparkle (Toe Pain).'

Learn from each experience as it will enhance future treatments.

Making the Abdominal Tapestry

Once the prescription has been decided upon, mark the points out and take note of the all the important landmarks such as Ren 9 (Shuifen), Ren 7 (Yinjiao) St 25 (Tianshu), etc. These points will act as the skeleton, upon which everything else is attached.

> **Tip:** Your prescription should serve as a scaffold only. Each treatment should be just like scaffolding in China where they use bamboo because it is flexible and can sway in typhoons rather than metal that is rigid, unforgiving and more likely to collapse!

Your prescription should allow for fluidity and intuition. Sometimes you might decide to use a point for no other reason than it feels right!

Build on these bones and add the flesh as you narrow the field and mark Ahshi points to treat a limb or a specific area of pain. See the patterns as mentioned in chapter 3, *Abdominal Point Location: Get to the Point*, before marking lots of different Ahshi points that will only serve to distort the bigger picture and confuse you. Once the main points are inserted and correct, then and only then should you isolate the painful Ahshi points.

> **Tip:** It is important to be precise. You should feel for Ahshi points in the areas where they are expected to be before needles are inserted. Needles around the affected area can change the picture and sometimes it is difficult to distinguish nodes from needle tips that are just superficially below the skin in the vicinity of where you are palpating. To avoid this get a mental picture of what is there from the start!

Keep it Simple

Why keep it simple? If treatment is for a shoulder problem, and you notice that there is an underlying Kidney Deficiency, this can be easily treated by combining the prescription 'Bringing Qi Home' and supplementing the Ren 4 (Guanyuan) with Kidney 13 (Qixue) points.

Always maintain focus and be disciplined. Only look for the problems that your client presents with and fix those issues before looking for other symptoms.

If, on palpating the abdomen, you notice a number of nodes and nodules in different areas, remember what your client has come to be treated for and avoid the temptation to start treating them for a pain in the ankle, head, lumbar area and the thumb! Otherwise, you will end up with a lot of unnecessary needles and an unfocused treatment that won't serve to improve your expertise or your reputation. Often more trivial problems will be corrected as your treatments progress and your client gets stronger.

Where? Why? When and How Deep?

Decide what your prescription is and locate all the points. If you need to add points think about each one and where the best Ahshi point will be found. For example, to treat the left medial knee the Ahshi point is most likely to be between the left knee points (Ab 4) and the medial knee point (Ab 5). If you are not getting a result at a particular Ahshi point ask yourself why, is the depth correct?

If the pain is in the Bone or deep in the joint, then the depth of the needle will be deeper than if it was at the skin or muscular level. If the pain is in a large area, then look at the option of using more needles. If the pain is in a line such as with sciatica moving from UB 40 (Weizhong) to UB 57 (Chengshan) then insert needles in a line between the knee point (Ab 4) to about halfway to the ankle point (Ab 6). The depth, in this case, will be deeper than if the problem was at the front of the leg but less deep than if the pain was in the buttock.

Remember, as you move down the limb the needles become more superficial. Adjust the depth until the desired result is achieved or until you instinctively know you are at the correct place.

Not all treatments will bear fruit immediately so be confident with your level of expertise; your client should feel the benefit within a day or two! Add more needles as you need but, always think **where, why and how deep?** Each needle should be logically thought out.

Outcome of Treatment

The outcome of each treatment is important and careful note-taking will help with future treatment and will show which treatments are most successful. With practice and the benefit of good case histories you can refine your skills and be more specific and minimalist if necessary.

Always highlight the results achieved with your clients so that they recognise the overall improvements as they happen. Clients are more likely to talk about you if you can show them that their pain has gone from an initial score of 10 down to 2, which is an 80% improvement, or, even better, that their pain has completely gone. Capitalise on these results and have your clients refer more clients by reminding them that a needle in the abdomen has fixed their pain.

If you are supplementing the abdominal treatment with traditional acupuncture treatment, it is always good to show clients the difference in needle sensation between abdominal acupuncture and the sensation of Qi they experience at points such as LI 4 (Hegu) or GB 34 (Yanglinguan). In my experience, most clients prefer the gentle nature of abdominal acupuncture.

Summary of Topics Covered in this Chapter

You can now put it all together in a methodical, logical and fluid fashion to cater for whatever painful conditions your clients should present. Here's how:

- Ask yourself, what's the problem?
- Where is the problem/pain likely to be reflected on the abdomen?

- Stick to the main issues that your client has come to you with.
- Look at what the abdomen is telling you
- Make a reference score for each pain!
- What is the treatment plan?
- Build on the scaffolding
- Get feedback as you needle Ahshi points
- Keep it simple
- Think it all through, needle, position, depth, function, etc.

Now that you have mastered the art of abdominal acupuncture go forth, practice, refine and learn from each treatment and every client. As I said at the beginning of this book, AA has changed my life and my practice. I hope it will change yours too.

If you need any further support with AA, please feel free to contact me at **dave@centre-force.ie** or subscribe to my Facebook page:
https://www.facebook.com/MasteringTheArtOfAbdominalAcupuncture?ref=bookmarks
for regular updates.

If you feel you want some practical hands-on experience check out my website **www.dan-tien.ie/centreforce** for the next Mastering the art of Abdominal Acupuncture workshop.

Acknowledgments

I would like to thank all those who have contributed to this book either directly, by means of advice, support, feedback or critical analysis, or indirectly, regarding my journey to this point.

I have to include all the teachers and students past, present and future who have, and will no doubt continue, to challenge, educate and inspire me. There are too many to mention here though a special thank-you must be given to Dr. Yang Ju Yi, Dr. Richard Tan, and, of course, to Dr. Han Yan, without whom I might never have explored AA. I am truly thankful to her for sharing so generously her time, knowledge, patience and passion with me. I also want to thank Dr. Ryan Pedersen, who introduced me to imaging methods including Dr. Tan's systems. Ryan also provided me with support and encouragement as well as reading and critically reviewing the first draft of this book.

Additionally, I want to thank all the teachers who fuel the passion that stokes the fire of knowledge and research into this beautiful field of TCM.

I feel privileged to work in such a diverse world of Health. TCM has so many interesting facets and modalities that attract characters from all kinds of backgrounds and cultures who share a passion for this wonderful world of acupuncture.

A very special thanks must be given to my beautiful partner Anna Goodere. Anna tirelessly and fearlessly went through the drafts, picking up on any inconsistencies and advising me on the layout and various aspects of putting the information in a more structured and logical way. I know this was not easy for her as I had moments of defensiveness and reluctance in making changes. Anna, I see now how right you were (now you have it in print!).

My good friend and colleague Bartley O'Brien for his feedback, constructive criticism and encouragement throughout and for taking the time to read various drafts of the book!

For all the wonderful illustrations, I thank Fergus Byrne, who showed patience and intuition with each piece of art.

Thanks to Martina Kenny also for the help with illustrations and graphics.

Thank you to my brother Ed for the great cover design.

Thanks also to my friend Sue Cuss for her support and contributions, and to Paul Masterson for all the technical help throughout the process.

A special gratitude goes to Siobhan Colgan, who has worked with me for the last six months of the process. Siobhan has transformed the book through her wonderful advice on structure, content and style, copyediting, proofreading, etc.

References

Bo, Z. (1993), "The Importance of the Acupoints Shenque in the study of Abdominal Acupuncture,' *Journal of Beijing Traditional Chinese Medicine*, 4, pp. 13-14.

Chace, C. & Shima, M. (2010) 'Theoretical Considerations', *An Exposition on the Eight Extraordinary Vessels: Acupuncture, Alchemy, and Herbal Medicine*, Seattle, USA, Eastland Press, p. 20.

Chace, C. & Shima, M. (2010) 'Theoretical Considerations', *An Exposition on the Eight Extraordinary Vessels: Acupuncture, Alchemy, and Herbal Medicine*, Seattle, USA, Eastland Press, p. 27.

D'Alberto, A. and Kim, E. (2005), 'An interview with Zhiyun Bo, inventor of abdominal acupuncture (Fu Zhen) acupuncture', *Acupuncture Today*, vol. 6, issue. 8, August, www.acupuncturetoday.com (accessed 11th Nov 2011).

Dr. Keown, D. (2014), 'A Name But No Form', The Spark in the Machine: How the Science of Acupuncture Explains the Mysteries of Western Medicine, London, Singing Dragon, pp. 12-15.

Dr. Keown, D. (2014), 'The Spark of Life', The Spark in the Machine: How the Science of Acupuncture Explains the Mysteries of Western Medicine, London, Singing Dragon, p. 20.

Dr. Keown, D. (2014), 'Tai Yin (Greater Yin)', The Spark in the Machine: How the Science of Acupuncture Explains the Mysteries of Western Medicine, Singing Dragon, p. 198.

Deadman Peter, Mazin Al Khafaji with Kevin Baker. Manual of Acupuncture App. Journal of Chinese Medicine Publications Ltd., 2011.

Ellis, A., Wiseman, N., Boss, K., *Grasping the Wind* (1993), Brookline, MA, Paradigm Publications

Guo F, Ma. L, Gong L. Zhang H (2003) 50 cases of prolapsed lumbar intervertebral disc using abdominal acupuncture *Journal of Chinese Acupuncture*; 23, p. 145

Hadhazy, A. (2010), 'Think Twice: How the Gut's "Second Brain" Influences Mood and Well-Being', *Scientific American*, http://www.scientificamerican.com/article/gut-second-brain/ (accessed 09/04/2015)

Lore, R. (2005) 'Abdominal Acupuncture: A Contemporary Microsystem Using Classical Chinese inspiration', *Acupuncture and Classical Chinese Medicine*, (accessed 09/04/2015) http://acupunc.blogspot.de/2005/11/abdominal-acupuncture-article.html

Maciocia, G. (2005) The Functions of the Six Extraordinary Tang Organs, *The Foundations of Chinese Medicine, A comprehensive textbook for Acupuncturists and Herbalists,* London, Elsevier Churchill Livingstone, pp. 123-125.

Maciocia, G. (2005), The Functions of the Triple Burner, *The Foundations of Chinese Medicine, A comprehensive textbook for Acupuncturists and Herbalists,* London, Elesvier Churchill Livingstone, pp.211-212.

Maciocia, G. (2005), The Functions of the Points, *The Foundations of Chinese Medicine, A comprehensive textbook for Acupuncturists and Herbalists,* London, Elesvier Churchill Livingstone, pp.385-387, 430-432, 460-464.

Dr. Pedersen, R. M. DOM, L.Ac. (2002) A Students – Teachers Guide to Clinical Acupuncture (second edition), pp.36-37, 46, 76-77, 106-111. East Mountain Associates LLC.

Peluffo, E. (2014) 'Cosmological Origins of the Obverse-Reverse Zang Fu Pairing in Chinese Medicine,' *Chinese Medicine*, 5, pp. 270-276.

Reid, D.P. (2001), 'A Modern, Practical Approach to the Ancient Way, The Tao of Health, Sex & Longevity', London, Pocket Books, p. 146.

Reid, T. (2008), 'The Neglected Art of Channel Palpation', *The Chinese Medicine Times*, Vol 3, Issue 1 Spring.

Ryan, P. M.S. L.AC. (2009) 'A Comprehensive Introduction to Abdominal Acupuncture', *Acupuncture Today*, Vol. 10, Issue 9, September http://www.acupuncturetoday.com/mpacms/at/article.php?id=32045 (Accessed Nov 2011).

Shan Disorder TCM Term, N.D. Available from: http://theory.yinyanghouse.com/theory/chinese/unique_tcm_conditions#shandisorder [27 September 2015].

Shang, C. (2009), Vol. 6, Issue 1, 'Prospective Tests on Biological Models of Acupuncture', *Evidence Based Complementary and Alternative Medicine,* http://www.ncbi.nlm.nih.gov/pmc/articles/PMC2644274/ (accessed 09/04/2015).

Tan, R. (2007), 'Specific Conditions – Ankle Sprain', Acupuncture 1, 2, 3, Richard Tan, (pp 35-42)

Tuvla, S. (2012) 'The Sacred Turtle and the Ba Gua: Case Studies', *European Journal of Oriental Medicine*, Vo. 7, No.1.

Tuvla, S. (2008) 'Abdominal Acupuncture (Fu Zhen): Energetic and Clinical Applications', *Journal of Chinese Medicine*, No. 87 (pp. 16-18).

Wang, J. & Robertson, J. (2008) 'The Shao Yang (Lesser Yang) System', *Applied Channel Theory in Chinese Medicine: Wang Ju-Yi's Lectures on Channel Therapy*, Seattle, Eastland Press, p. 227.

Wang, J. & Robertson, J. (2008), Applied Channel Theory in Chinese Medicine: Wang Ju-Yi's Lectures on Channel Therapy, Seattle, Eastland Press, pp. 190-193.

Wang, J. (2013) Channel Theory (lecture to Trinity College, Dublin), 14 June.

Yang C, Acupuncture Microsystems and Advanced Treatment Techniques, Course Notes, University of Technology Sydney, Australia.2012. Last accessed 1/10/15.

Yang, L. (1998), *The Contemporary study of book of changes,* Book of Changes and Traditional Chinese Medicine, Beijing, Beijing Science and Technology Press, p.6.

Yang, L. (1998), *The Contemporary study of book of changes,* Book of Changes and Traditional Chinese Medicine, Beijing, Beijing Science and Technology Press, p.37.

Zhang, Z. (2013) *Jin Gui Yao Lue: Essential Prescriptions of the Golden Cabinet, Translation & Commentaries*, Seattle, Eastland Press.

Appendices

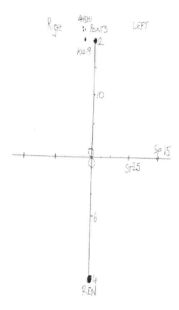

Fig A 1 Illustrates how to keep simple prescription notes. This is the precription for Discoteque dislocated Jaw (see pg 135)

Fig A 2 Illustrates simple prescription method for Normans neuralgia (see page 164)

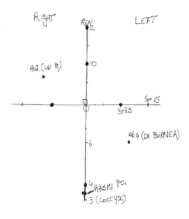

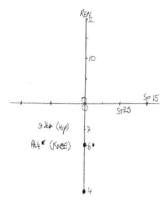

Fig A 3 Illustrates simple prescription method for Not for the Faint Hearted (see page 34)

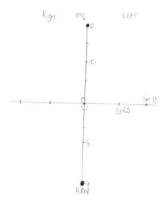

Fig A 4 Illustrates simple AA Prescription used for case history 'Needle Phobic with a Headache' (see page 126)

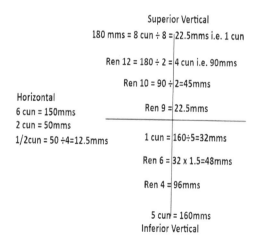

Superior Vertical

180 mms = 8 cun ÷ 8 = 22.5mms i.e. 1 cun

Ren 12 = 180 ÷ 2 = 4 cun i.e. 90mms

Ren 10 = 90 ÷2=45mms

Horizontal
6 cun = 150mms
2 cun = 50mms
1/2cun = 50 ÷4=12.5mms

Ren 9 = 22.5mms

1 cun = 160÷5=32mms

Ren 6 = 32 x 1.5=48mms

Ren 4 = 96mms

5 cun = 160mms
Inferior Vertical

Fig A 5 Illustrates the completed record sheet of AA point location using the example from the mathematical formulaic ruler method used in chapter 3

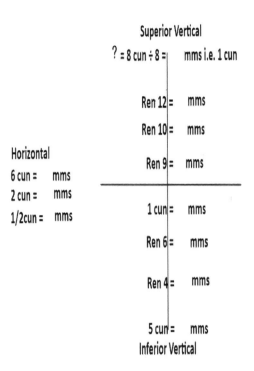

Superior Vertical

? = 8 cun ÷ 8 =   mms i.e. 1 cun

Ren 12 =   mms

Ren 10 =   mms

Horizontal

Ren 9 =   mms

6 cun =   mms

2 cun =   mms

1/2cun =   mms

1 cun =   mms

Ren 6 =   mms

Ren 4 =   mms

5 cun =   mms

Inferior Vertical

Fig A 6 An example of a blank record chart for the formulaic ruler measurment method

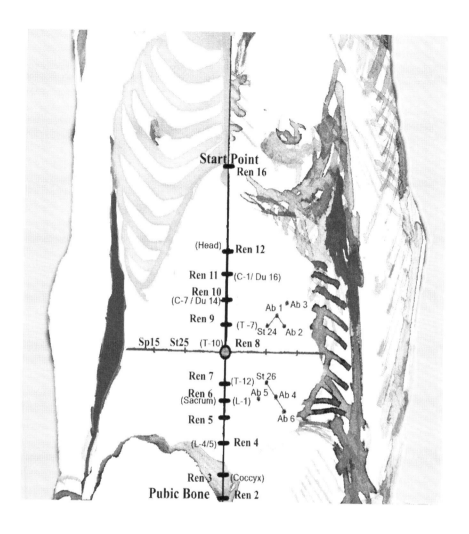

Start Point
Ren 16

(Head) Ren 12

Ren 11 (C-1/ Du 16)
Ren 10 (C-7 / Du 14)

Ren 9
(T -7) St 24 Ab 2
Ab 1 Ab 3

Sp15 St25 (T-10) Ren 8

Ren 7 (T-12) St 26
Ren 6 (L-1) Ab 5 Ab 4
(Sacrum)
Ren 5 Ab 6

(L-4/5) Ren 4

Ren 3 (Coccyx)
Pubic Bone Ren 2

Fig A 7 The anatomical importance of the main AA points with limb patterns

~ 325 ~

Quick Reference Chart highlighting AA Ren points

Abdominal Acupuncture Point	Turtle Anatomical area of significance	Location	Heaven level indications
Ren 12 (Zhongwan)	Mouth	4 cun superior to Ren 8 (Shenque)	Mouth, head, face.
Ren 11 (Jianli)	Upper throat / Du 16 (Fengfu)	3 cun superior to Ren 8 (Shenque)	Throat and cervical vertebrae No.1
Ren 10 (Xiawan)	Lower throat / Du 14 (Dazhui)	2 cun superior to Ren 8 (Shenque)	Lower aspect of the neck cervical vertebra No.7
Ren 9 (Shuifen)	Level with 7th thoracic vertebrae (T-7).	1 cun superior to Ren 8 (Shenque)	Mid back or chest pain. Landmark for St 24 (Huaroumen)

Ren 8 (Shenque)	Level with 10th thoracic vertebrae (T-10).	In the centre of umbilicus (never needle)	Either side treats back pain at T-10.
Ren 7	Level with 12th thoracic vertebrae (T-12).	1 cun inferior to Ren 8 (Shenque)	Pain of 12th vertebra landmark for St 26 (Wailing).
Ren 6 (Qihai)	Level with lumbar vertebrae no.1 (L-1)	1.5 cun inferior to Ren 8 (Shenque)	Lumbar pain around L-1. Pelvic or groin pain.
Ren 4 (Guanyuan)	Level with lumbar vertebrae no.4 or 5 (L-4 or 5)	3 cun inferior to Ren 8 (Shenque)	Lumbar pain around L-4 or 5. Pelvic or groin pain.

Table A 1. Summary of the Ren points area of influence at the heaven level. (Yang C. 2012)

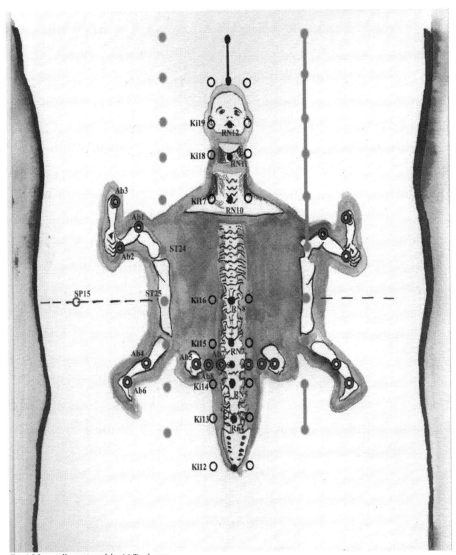

Fig A 8 Large illustration of the AA Turtle map

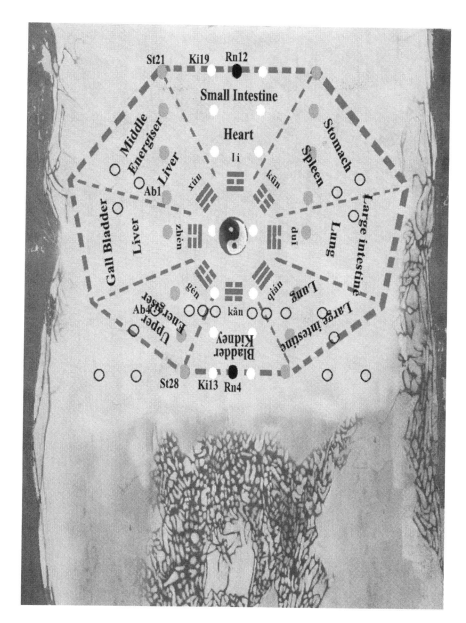

Fig A 9 Enlarged Illustration of the AA Ba Gua

INDEX

prescription, 40, 111, 125, 134, 162, 167, 169, 172, 182, 183, 184, 185, 186, 190, 197, 210, 213, 216, 227, 232, 234, 236, 246, 247, 250, 253, 254, 258, 263, 265, 266, 268, 270, 274, 275, 278, 279, 280, 289, 290, 291, 292, 293, 296, 298, 299, 301, 302, 303, 304, 306, 311, 312, 313, 321, 322

prescriptions, 1, 20, 65, 68, 179, 201, 202, 204, 205, 221, 287, 303, 304, 306

Professor Zhiyun Bo, 19, 24, 246

prognosis, 160, 298

protocol, 108, 163, 213, 236, 241, 249, 262

pubic bone, 77, 83, 100, 123

pulse, 17, 26, 153, 154, 236, 265, 298

Qi, 19, 40, 41, 42, 43, 44, 48, 50, 52, 54, 56, 58, 59, 60, 61, 63, 64, 65, 66, 111, 112, 113, 115, 116, 117, 119, 121, 122, 125, 126, 127, 128, 130, 134, 136, 137, 138, 139, 140, 141, 143, 144, 148, 150, 151, 154, 156, 157, 158, 159, 160, 161, 169, 171, 172, 174, 179, 180, 181, 182, 183, 185, 189, 190, 191, 197, 203, 205, 207, 209, 210, 211, 213, 216, 220, 221, 223, 225, 227, 229, 232, 234, 236, 240, 242, 249, 251, 254, 257, 260, 261, 262, 264, 265, 268, 272, 273, 275, 277, 279, 282, 285, 288, 289, 291, 293, 296, 298, 301, 303, 310, 312, 314

Qi Gong, 40, 56

Qi Nei Zang, 40

Qian, 48, 52, 150, 192

quadratus lumborum, 139, 243

radiating pain, 254

record charts, 304

records, 89, 304

rectus abdominis, 142

reduction, 26, 31, 33, 169, 257, 258, 259, 264, 286

reference point score, 224, 264, 270

reference score, 173, 256, 309, 315

referred pain, 215, 253

regular channels, 61

Ren 1(Huiyin), 162

Ren 10 (Xiawan), 27, 79, 87, 88, 92, 93, 104, 105, 111, 116, 117, 118, 162, 180, 181, 189, 206, 207, 208, 209, 210, 213, 216, 220, 223, 234, 242, 249, 257, 260, 265, 275, 279, 282, 289, 296, 298, 326

Ren 11 (Jianli), 27, 64, 92, 114, 115, 117, 206, 210, 296, 326

Ren 12 (Zhongwan), 24, 27, 63, 64, 65, 78, 79, 91, 92, 111, 112, 113, 115, 117, 118, 124, 125, 134, 157, 160, 162, 177, 180, 181, 182, 183, 189, 195, 197, 205, 207, 210, 211, 213, 216, 217, 218, 220, 223, 224, 226, 227, 230, 232, 234, 236, 238, 242, 249, 254, 257, 260, 265, 268, 272, 275, 279, 280, 282, 285, 289, 296, 298, 299, 301, 326

Ren 3 (Zhongji), 56, 123, 126, 127, 162, 243

Ren 4 (Guanyuan), 24, 27, 33, 39, 52, 56, 65, 83, 100, 101, 107, 111, 122, 123, 124, 125, 128, 129, 132, 134, 151, 157, 159, 160, 161, 162, 166, 170, 180, 181, 182, 183, 189, 195, 196, 197, 203, 210, 213, 216, 217, 220, 223, 224, 230, 232, 234, 238, 240, 242, 243, 245, 246, 247, 249, 251, 252, 254, 257, 260, 261, 265, 268, 272, 273, 275, 279, 280, 282, 283, 285, 289, 296, 298, 301, 304, 312, 327

Ren 5 (Shimen), 60

Ren 6 (Qihai), 27, 33, 39, 52, 56, 65, 83, 84, 85, 101, 103, 107, 111, 121, 122, 125, 146, 166, 180, 181, 189, 195, 196, 197, 203, 210, 213, 216, 220, 223, 229, 232, 234, 242, 243, 245, 246, 247, 249, 251, 252, 254, 257, 260, 265, 268, 272, 273, 275, 279, 282, 283, 289, 296, 298, 301, 304, 327

Ren 7 (Yinjiao), 77, 83, 84, 85, 100, 107, 120, 139, 239, 302, 311

Ren 8 (Shenque), 37, 41, 42, 43, 44, 55, 57, 61, 67, 78, 79, 80, 82, 98, 113, 115, 117, 118, 119, 122, 138, 156, 157, 159, 161, 217, 218, 239, 309, 326, 327

Ren 9 (Shuifen), 27, 60, 77, 79, 87, 93, 94, 104, 117, 118, 136, 161, 170, 204, 206, 210, 213, 218, 236, 239, 240, 242, 245, 247, 249, 251, 254, 260, 261, 272, 283, 310, 311, 326

Ren Mai, 39, 61, 62, 64, 67, 113, 121, 158, 243

repetitive strain injury, 215, 305

resistance, 117, 161, 166, 172, 173, 174, 203, 210, 225, 243, 264, 290

16226863R00181

Printed in Great Britain
by Amazon